MW01122773

Resident's Guide to Treatment of People With Chronic Mental Illness

Committee on Psychiatry and the Community
Group for the Advancement of Psychiatry
(Participants in the preparation of this report)

Kenneth Minkoff, Woburn, MA, *Chairperson*
C. Knight Aldrich, Charlottesville, VA
Leona Bachrach, Gaithersburg, MD
Stephen Goldfinger, Boston, MA
David G. Greenfeld, Guilford, CT
H. Richard Lamb, Los Angeles, CA,
John C. Nemiah, Hanover, NH
Becky Potter, Tucson, AZ
Alexander S. Rogawski, Los Angeles, CA
John J. Schwab, Louisville, KY
John A. Talbott, Baltimore, MD
Allan Tasman, Louisville, KY
Charles B. Wilkinson, Kansas City, MO

Stephen Jarvis, Kansas City, MO *(GAP Fellow)*
Linda M. Peterson, Owings Mills, MD *(GAP Fellow)*
Kimberly Yonkers, Belmont, MA *(GAP Fellow)*

Resident's Guide to Treatment of People With Chronic Mental Illness

Formulated by the
Committee on Psychiatry
and the Community

Group for the Advancement of Psychiatry

Report No. 136

Published by

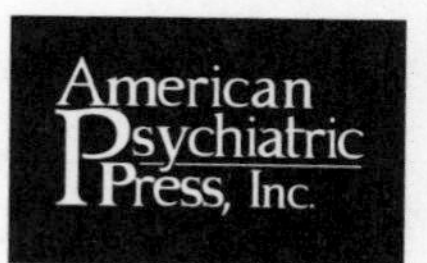

Washington, DC
London, England

Manufactured in the United States of America on acid-free paper
96 4 3 2
Published by American Psychiatric Press, Inc.
1400 K Street, N.W., Washington, DC 20005

Library of Congress Cataloging-in-Publication Data

Resident's guide to treatment of people with chronic mental illness / formulated by the Committee on Psychiatry and the Community, Group for the Advancement of Psychiatry.
p. cm. — (Report : no. 136)
Includes bibliographical references and index.
ISBN (invalid) 08713182049 (alk. paper)
1. Mentally ill—Treatment. 2. Chronically ill—Treatment. 3. Psychiatry—Study and teaching (Residency). I. Group for the Advancement of Psychiatry. Committee on Psychiatry and Community. II. Series: Report (Group for the Advancement of Psychiatry : 1984) : no. 136.
[DNLM: 1. Chronic Diseases. 2. Mental disorders—therapy. W1 RE209BR no. 136 / WM 400 R433]
RC321.G7 no. 136
[RC480.53]
616.89'1]
[616.89'1]
DNLM/DLC 92-48698
for Library of Congress CIP

British Library Cataloguing in Publication Data

A CIP record is available from the British Library.

This report is dedicated to the memory of
Alexander S. Rogawski and Charles B. Wilkinson,
whose invaluable contributions
have added so much in so many ways
to the Group for the Advancement of Psychiatry,
to the Committee on Psychiatry and the Community,
and to the publication of this report.

Contents

Foreword: A Resident's Perspective

My introduction to this guidebook for residents occurred well before it found its way to print. As a third-year resident, I was awarded one of the Group for the Advancement of Psychiatry's Ginsburg Fellowships, and the committee to which I was assigned had recently begun work on this guidebook. For 3 years I participated both in learning more about the treatment of chronically mentally ill patients and in writing this guide.

During these years I found that my views about treating chronically mentally ill patients evolved in ways that surprised me. I had not come to the committee with any special skills in working with this group of patients; my training program put less emphasis on working with them than it did on working with other patient groups. Although psychopharmacological issues were addressed, little was taught about how to talk to or conduct therapy with chronic patients, an omission which my colleagues and I found particularly frustrating, because we had many schizophrenic patients both as inpatients and outpatients. At times we wondered if, perhaps, the simple truth was that there really was not much that we as physicians could do for these patients.

I therefore joined the committee with a good deal of skepticism, but over the next 3 years my point of view changed considerably. Through the process of developing this guidebook, many of my questions about the comprehensive treatment of chronically mentally ill patients have been answered. Moreover, I have come to realize that the psychotherapeutic treatment of these patients can be just as elegant and challenging as therapy with other patients. Knowing how to work with them makes their care more satisfying as well as more interesting, which is one of the reasons why this guide is so valuable—for residents and for other mental health practitioners.

In this guidebook we describe the direct involvement of psychiatric residents in a broad range of treatment interventions. Some residents may prefer to read the guide cover to cover, while others may prefer using it when a particular clinical situation arises, referring to specific topics in the table of contents or index. No matter how the book is used, it can be a valuable resource for residents and other mental health professionals working with this population. For me, the skills and interventions explored in this book have been useful not only during my residency but also with patients I have continued to treat since then.

Introduction

One significant barrier to the provision of high-quality services to persons with chronic mental illness has been the lack of adequate clinical training in treating this population. The GAP Committee on Psychiatry and the Community became interested in this problem during the course of working on our previous report, in which we reviewed numerous letters from family members commenting on the difficulty of locating a psychiatrist who was informed and interested in the treatment of long-term mental illness.[1] As a consequence, we surveyed a group of psychiatric residents and gathered a list of over 30 clinical questions faced by residents treating this population. This book was written specifically to attempt to answer those questions.

Virtually all residents are perplexed and apprehensive when they begin to treat patients with chronic mental illness. Although many of their questions may be answered as training proceeds, and much of their apprehension allayed, this process takes time, and many residents "burn out" trying to treat chronically mentally ill patients long before they learn how to do it. Moreover, in many training programs, resources for training residents to treat this population are so limited that residents never feel adequately trained at all.

The purpose of this book is to help residents—and other beginning clinicians—to gain a basic understanding of the clinical principles and techniques that underlie therapeutic work with patients who have chronic mental illness and with their families. Our focus in this guide is neither theoretical nor abstract, but practical, and the emphasis is on interpersonal interventions rather than on specific psychopharmacological prescriptions. We will illustrate specific techniques, including the use of supervision (the book is intended to supplement—not replace—individual clinical supervision), for dealing with a range of clinical situations by using case examples and clinical vignettes that reflect our own experiences and the experiences of our colleagues and trainees. Through these specific examples and techniques, we hope not only to answer residents' questions about how to work with this population but also to convey two important messages: 1) persons with

---

[1]Group for the Advancement of Psychiatry: *A Family Affair: Helping Families Cope With Mental Illness—A Guide for the Professions* (GAP Report No. 119). New York, Brunner/Mazel, 1986.

chronic mental illness can benefit from interpersonal treatment methods, and 2) this population of patients can be enormously rewarding to treat.

In Chapter 1 we introduce the reader to three patients and their doctors in three typical residency settings: the emergency room, the inpatient unit, and the outpatient clinic. We then describe a theoretical framework governing the overall strategy of assessment and treatment that is illustrated as these and other patients and residents are revisited in the following chapters.

In the next section of the book (Chapters 2–4) we discuss engagement and assessment. In Chapter 2 we describe the initial steps of assessing patients and engaging them in treatment. Because the family is an integral part of the treatment, we use a separate chapter (Chapter 3) to discuss the inclusion of the family in such treatment. Similar principles are applied to the treatment system in Chapter 4.

In the next section of the book (Chapters 5–9) we address treatment. In Chapter 5 we present a model for formulating treatment plans, and in Chapter 6 we discuss the implementation of those plans with regard to pharmacological interventions. In Chapter 7, in which the "nuts and bolts" of individual therapy are discussed, the committee considers basic questions about the structure of therapy and offers examples from therapy sessions. Our task in Chapter 8, in relation to the individual therapy discussed in Chapter 7, is to focus on therapy with the family. In Chapter 9, we discuss ways to mobilize community resources in the treatment of chronically mentally ill patients.

In the final section of the book we discuss the treatment of special populations, specifically patients with dual diagnosis of major mental illness and substance use disorders (Chapter 10), and homeless mentally ill patients (Chapter 11). Specific assessment tools and a selected reading list are included at the end of the book.

Note that several of the case vignettes continue through more than one chapter. Although this may at times be confusing, we believe that it is an important way for the reader to experience how the assessment and treatment of patients unfold in longitudinal fashion. To help the reader keep track of the cases, we have included a case index that indicates where each case is first discussed and where it is subsequently mentioned.

All patient and physician names in this manual are fictitious.

1

Baptism of Fire

A Tour of the Front: Three Clinical Vignettes

Emergency Room

Mary Hogarth[1]

On a late afternoon toward the end of August, nearly 2 months into her first year of psychiatric residency in a general hospital, Dr. Holt is facing her weekly night on call. Her colleagues have finished their work, and the daytime emergency room (ER) resident turns the emergency beeper over to her. She is on her way to the dining room, wondering a bit apprehensively what the night ahead will bring, when she is paged by the ER.

Over the phone the psychiatric triage clinician sounds urgent and a bit disgusted as he tells her that Mary Hogarth has just been brought in—again! He insists that Dr. Holt come to the ER right away, explaining that the patient has been brought from the sheltered workshop by two security guards after having a "fit," and is now agitated and uncooperative. He has called the workshop to find out what happened, but all the staff, including the patient's case manager, had left for the day.

Dr. Holt takes a deep breath; she can feel her apprehension rise. She has a momentary urge to call her senior backup but dismisses the thought; she knows that now that she has been through several nights on call, he will expect her at least to make a preliminary examination

---

[1]For continuation of this case study, see pp. 17–18, 30, 59, 62–63, 72–74, 81–82, 109, and 142.

on her own before consulting him. She doesn't want to become known as a weak link in the system, yet she still wishes that she wasn't alone with the Mary Hogarth problem.

Many questions race through Dr. Holt's mind as she walks down to the ER. Why was the clinician so insistent—and so negative? Was it because the patient is violent or out of control? Or is it that Mary Hogarth is a well-known "chronic" who "abuses the system"? Is there a treatment plan for her that I should know about? Should I talk to the patient alone, or would it be wise to keep a security guard with us? What am I going to say to the patient? If she is agitated, how am I going to calm her down? Dr. Holt envisions the security guards holding down an infuriated and struggling patient, still irrational after having attacked her colleagues at her workplace. Dr. Holt hopes her backup is still in the house.

As Dr. Holt arrives in the ER, the triage clinician hands her the chart, commenting, "This is the fourth time she's been here in the last 3 months. She's always looking for attention. What she needs is a trip to the state hospital—that'll teach her a lesson!" He points to a room with a security guard outside the door.

Glancing briefly into the room, Dr. Holt sees a disheveled and agitated young woman pacing up and down, gesticulating vigorously and answering what appear to be hallucinatory voices. The woman looks as if she is ready to strike out at any moment, and Dr. Holt wonders if the patient should be restrained. However, she is not sure that, in or out of restraints, the patient will be able to determine what is going on.

Dr. Holt notices a distraught older woman, apparently the patient's mother, standing by the nursing-station counter and tearfully wringing her hands as she holds the nurse by the arm. With difficulty the nurse detaches herself from the mother's grasp and, with an impatient look, approaches Dr. Holt. She tells Dr. Holt that the patient will not talk about what has happened but only mumbles that she will "get revenge on the people who have been killing small children throughout the country."

Because it seems obvious that the patient cannot give a valid history herself, Dr. Holt decides to talk to the mother first. The mother confirms what the nurse had just said and adds that the patient had been staying up all night for a week, ruminating aloud about the murders her supervisor and co-workers at the workshop had allegedly masterminded. The mother is perplexed and confused, and cannot identify any precipitants for this behavior. On the one hand she is worried and knows that something is dreadfully wrong, but on the other hand she tries desperately to convince Dr. Holt that her daughter is not seriously ill. "Mary was in a psychiatric hospital several years ago and has never been the same since," she says. "It must have been the hospital that made her sick; I don't want her to go through that ordeal again. Mary takes a lot of different pills; maybe the pills are making her crazy. Can't you just give her a shot of something to calm her down, so I can take her home?"

Despite the mother's request, Dr. Holt does not believe that she can allow the patient to leave, especially since the patient has been brought in by the security police and may well have homicidal thoughts. Seeing that she may have to persuade Mrs. Hogarth to agree to Mary's hospitalization, Dr. Holt is not sure exactly how to proceed.

To help with this question, Dr. Holt decides to ask the triage clinician how Ms. Hogarth had been dealt with in the past. "There's nothing you can do," says the clinician disgustedly. "Either commit her and get it over with, or give her some medication to calm her down, and then send her home as we did the last time. But if you do, she'll be back next week."

Dr. Holt feels annoyed at the clinician's negative attitude, but is not sure that she is not being naive to think that such a chronic patient might respond to a more positive approach. She would like to see what would happen if Ms. Hogarth were to have a period of stabilization on the university hospital inpatient unit, but that would require the patient to agree to go into the hospital voluntarily.

Dr. Holt soon realizes that she can temporize no longer—she must talk to the patient now in order to work out a plan of action. But how is she to deal with the violent agitation? She recalls something she picked up at a clinical conference: to calm down agitated patients, try to make them physically and emotionally comfortable by, for example, offering them a drink or food. She decides to try this strategy; keeping the security guard at her side, she enters the patient's room.

To her surprise and relief, the patient responds to Dr. Holt's offer of a can of ginger ale and sits down quietly. "So far, so good," Dr. Holt thinks, "but how can I get her to tell me what is troubling her without getting her agitated again?" Dr. Holt remembers what ward patients have told her about their ER experiences—how confused and frightened and suspicious they felt in the face of all that was going on around them, and how difficult it was to talk about what was troubling them.

Dr. Holt knows that she needs detailed information from her patient about her recent behavior and her inner perceptions and fears. She is also aware that the initial contact with a patient is vital for establishing the therapeutic relationship that will facilitate treatment on the inpatient unit. How should she proceed? What should she say and do?

Dr. Holt's concerns are not unique. This vignette reflects common problems experienced by psychiatric residents and other beginning clinicians when learning to treat chronically psychotic patients. Before discussing the answers to these questions regarding the management of Mary Hogarth, we will describe two additional problem situations that residents may face—one on the psychiatric inpatient unit, and the other in the outpatient clinic.

Inpatient Unit

The majority of patients on teaching-hospital psychiatric units are acutely ill, and most respond quickly to treatment. Occasionally, however, a patient is admitted with a relatively long history of psychiatric hospitalization, as in the following example:

Matthew Jermyn[2]

Matthew Jermyn has been a "revolving-door patient"—that is, he has been repeatedly hospitalized, released, and rehospitalized during the course of his illness. This time, Mr. Jermyn has only been out of the hospital a few months, living in his parents' home and leading a marginal existence. As usual, he stopped taking his prescribed medication shortly after his discharge and has now relapsed.

Mr. Jermyn is not received on the ward with enthusiasm, and beneath the staff's professional veneer there is an underlying irritation. If only he had continued taking his medication, they would have been spared the nuisance of admitting him. Compliance is the issue: if he takes his medication, he will stay out of the hospital; if he does not, he will be back again.

The resident, Dr. Transome, knows that an important goal of hospitalization is to get Mr. Jermyn to continue to take his medication after he leaves the hospital. What can he say to convince his patient of the absolute necessity to comply with treatment? Should he try to form a relationship with Mr. Jermyn—or would it be a waste of time? Mr. Jermyn's behavior is irrational and his train of thought is hard to follow. For example, when he asks to leave the hospital, he gives as his reason that the other half of him lives in New York City. "People," he says, "consider me to be Jesus Christ. Don't you know, Doctor, the demons are leaving my body through my belly button?"

Dr. Transome not only finds communication with Mr. Jermyn difficult, but he feels frightened by the patient's angry stare and his threatening posture. He wonders what he should say when Mr. Jermyn stands uncomfortably close to him and gesticulates. Is Mr. Jermyn about to lose control? Does he need more medication or even restraint? "Maybe I should just avoid him till the meds start to work," thinks Dr. Transome. "I can't think of anything to say to calm him down." Should he try to interpret the patient's thoughts or correct his misperceptions, or should he make comments that are supportive and concrete?

The staff psychiatrist, the nurses, and Dr. Transome's fellow residents all tell him that he is wasting his time trying to accomplish

---

[2]For continuation of this case study, see pp. 32, 38–39, 43–44, 49, 57–58, 65, 80–81, 83, 92–93, 98, 100–101, 119, 120–121, and 141–142.

anything with Mr. Jermyn. The only real issue, they insist, is whether the patient should be started on depot medication. Dr. Transome is less fatalistic and wonders if, with time and effort, he could persuade Mr. Jermyn to comply with the plan for oral medication. He perceives, however, that Mr. Jermyn is dispirited by his chronic illness and that he has almost given up. He recognizes that Mr. Jermyn's despair is well founded and that changing this attitude would probably require time-consuming psychotherapeutic interventions.

Meanwhile, Dr. Transome's schedule is full and his time must be rationed. Furthermore, even if he devotes time to Mr. Jermyn, progress will be slow at best. Besides, his other patients are less bizarre, more communicative, and less frightening. Perhaps everyone else is right. Dr. Transome begins to think that it would be easier to treat Mr. Jermyn as expeditiously as possible, freeing up his time and energy for patients considered more therapeutically "rewarding."

Dr. Transome's one brief meeting with Mr. Jermyn's parents is not a success. In the meeting, the patient's parents plead with Dr. Transome to transfer their son to a state hospital when his stay on the general hospital psychiatric ward is up, or at least not to send him home for a few weeks so that they may have some respite from caring for him. Dr. Transome feels caught in the middle. From his patient's behavior on the ward Dr. Transome can well imagine what it must be like for Mr. Jermyn's parents to have him at home; at the same time, he knows that the state hospital would discharge him in a few days. To add to his dilemma, he is under pressure from the attending psychiatrist to send Mr. Jermyn home quickly. Beset on all sides, Dr. Transome feels overwhelmed and cuts the interview short.

Mr. Jermyn refuses the recommendation for depot medication, promising not very convincingly that in the future he will take his pills faithfully. With oral medication, he soon becomes less psychotic and more manageable. Convinced that his patient's psychosis is chronic and discouraged about his patient's future course, Dr. Transome plans to schedule Mr. Jermyn for a follow-up appointment in the medication clinic with another resident, thinking "I'm glad I'm not the one who has to follow him." He also plans to avoid Mr. Jermyn's family when they come to take their son home. But as the time of Mr. Jermyn's discharge approaches, Dr. Transome continues to wonder whether there is anything else he can do or say to achieve a more successful outcome. He feels uncomfortable about this disposition.

As we can see, Dr. Transome's tasks are similar to those that confront Dr. Holt. Both residents face the immediate problem of performing an accurate clinical assessment despite serious difficulties with communication. Both residents are challenged to establish a therapeutic relationship and to develop a treatment plan for a difficult and resistant patient. And in both instances the residents have to proceed in the face of conflicting attitudes and demands from their colleagues and members of the patients' families.

Successful treatment for each patient is likely to require the development of a long-term treatment plan aimed not only at the individual patient's specific clinical problem but at family members' needs as well, enhancing their ability to provide adequate social and emotional support. In each case the plan requires more than simple prescriptions of medication.

Outpatient Clinic

The situation in an outpatient clinic can provide different challenges for the physician, as in the following example:

Ms. DeBarry[3]

Dr. Lyon is just beginning his outpatient rotation. As he reviews the chart of his first patient, he remembers how the senior resident, while signing off her cases, rolled her eyes in mock despair when reaching Ms. DeBarry, saying, sarcastically, "Here's a 'good' psychotherapy patient for you." She told him that the patient had a chronic "rapid cycling bipolar disorder."

Dr. Lyon goes to the waiting room to find Ms. DeBarry sitting calmly, reading a magazine. He introduces himself and invites Ms. DeBarry into his office. He begins the session by commenting that he knows a little about her from her previous psychiatrist. Ms. DeBarry interrupts to inform Dr. Lyon that she has very complicated psychiatric problems, including "rapid cycling bipolar disorder, bulimia, and a variant of obsessive-compulsive disorder." She goes on to name five of the top psychiatrists in the city with whom she has had consultations to confirm these diagnoses. She informs Dr. Lyon that the effective treatment of her illness has eluded all those who have preceded him, and she sees no reason to think that he will fare any better.

Dr. Lyon's head is spinning. Although he is well aware of the existence and nature of these disorders, he has not yet treated anyone suffering from them. He begins to wonder how he can manage a patient who has had so many clinical problems and who has seen so many well-known psychiatrists without benefit. In the face of their failures, how is he to elicit the patient's trust and engage her in treatment?

Ms. DeBarry continues. She lists for Dr. Lyon all the medications she has tried, including many of which he has not heard. She informs

[3]For continuation of this case study, see pp. 81, 102, 109, 112, and 143.

him that she knows best what she needs and names a new antidepressant that Dr. Lyon has never used. She urges him to call her former psychiatrist, who "really knew her, truly understood her, and was available to her any hour of the day or night."

Although Dr. Lyon is sure that this colleague is interested in all of his patients, he doubts that he tolerated being constantly available, day and night. He suspects that Ms. DeBarry will require "limit setting," but he is not sure whether the first session is the appropriate time to initiate such a restriction or whether it may drive the patient away. Although he is certain that he does not want to be called any hour of the day or night, he is not sure just where to set the limits.

Dr. Lyon is curious about Ms. DeBarry's previous psychiatrist. She speaks about him in glowing terms, yet claims that he had not "effectively" treated her complicated problems. Dr. Lyon suspects that Ms. DeBarry harbors an "idealizing," and even an eroticized, transference to her former psychiatrist. Will the patient's longing for her previous therapist make it difficult for her to develop a therapeutic rapport with Dr. Lyon? When should he address the patient's change of therapist—now, later, or never?

As could be predicted from the first meeting, difficult problems in Ms. DeBarry's treatment arose almost immediately. At the end of the first session the patient left with instructions to continue her medications as previously prescribed and to return in a week. Three days later Ms. DeBarry telephoned Dr. Lyon to inform him that, although she had not mentioned it during her first visit, she had in fact stopped taking her medications the week before attending the clinic. She now reports that she feels terrible, is confused, and thinks people may be plotting to harm her. She has barely slept for the past two nights and thinks she needs to come into the hospital.

Ms. DeBarry sounds so distressed that Dr. Lyon makes an appointment for that afternoon to evaluate her for admission, but she fails to appear. When Dr. Lyon telephones her home, her mother tells him that the patient is out and then angrily asks why he told her daughter to stop taking her medication. She refuses to accept Dr. Lyon's version of the events, telling him that psychiatrists only want their patients' money.

Despite her anger, the mother is obviously concerned about her daughter, but her response to Dr. Lyon's further questioning makes it clear that she knows little about her daughter's illness. Worried about the potential for suicidal behavior in a patient he does not know well, Dr. Lyon suggests alerting the police to the fact that she is missing. The mother adamantly rejects the idea and hangs up.

In a quandary, Dr. Lyon tries to reach his supervisor for advice, but before the supervisor returns his call, the patient telephones. She apologizes for missing the appointment but says that she took some pills and was finally able to fall asleep at a friend's house. She tells Dr.

> Lyon that she would like to come in tomorrow to talk with him. She promises to take her medication as prescribed, no longer wants to be admitted to the hospital, and promises not to do anything to hurt herself.

Dr. Lyon is uncertain. Shouldn't Ms. DeBarry be in the hospital where she can be watched closely? Although she has said she would not harm herself, Dr. Lyon is uneasy, for the patient has already been misleading in her failure to reveal that she had stopped taking her medication. Can Dr. Lyon believe anything she says? Can he be confident that she is safe?

Although he has seen Ms. DeBarry only once, he still wonders uneasily whether he might have done more. Should he have said something else or have outlined a more specific treatment plan, or arranged to include family members in the patient's management? And what *is* the treatment plan anyway? Is he supposed to do psychotherapy with Ms. DeBarry, and if so, how? From what he has learned of psychotherapy thus far, it consists mainly of sitting calmly in an office while the patient "free-associates." How would that work with such a chaotic patient as Ms. DeBarry? And yet, because she seems to have a personality disorder as well as an affective illness, he suspects that medication alone will not be enough to help her. What approach can Dr. Lyon take?

Three Clinical Settings, One Set of Clinical Dilemmas

Dr. Lyon faces a similar problem in the outpatient clinic to those faced by Drs. Holt and Transome: the treatment of a patient in an acute crisis that has arisen during the course of a chronic mental illness. Situations like those in the vignettes are common in residency training, because most patients with chronic mental illness have episodes of acute exacerbation separated by longer periods of relative stability. For a beginning resident, the clinical needs of such patients can be extraordinarily complicated and anxiety provoking.

These three patients present their respective clinicians with challenging tasks, as outlined in Table 1–1. The first tasks confronting Dr. Holt, for example, are to establish communication with a frightened, paranoid patient; to reassure her equally distressed mother; and to allay the anxieties of an apprehensive emergency room staff. Once she calms these troubled waters, Dr. Holt can turn to the larger task of establishing a diagnosis and instituting a treatment plan that will include active supportive measures for both the patient and her mother.

Table 1–1. Initial tasks for treatment of chronically mentally ill patients

Ensure patient and clinician safety.
Make an accurate diagnosis, often despite serious barriers to establishing communication and to forming an empathic connection.
Develop a treatment relationship, often with a resistant, provocative, bizarre, and chronically disturbed individual.
Engage involved, although often difficult and resistant, family members whose anxieties and demands compound an already difficult situation.
Implement an immediate treatment plan to defuse an acute crisis safely.
Formulate a plan to help the patient maintain control of the illness and prevent future exacerbations.
Formulate a long-range plan to help the patient and family — to acknowledge, accept, and bear the painful reality of living within the limits imposed by a chronic illness. — to learn to make slow progress within those limits by participation in rehabilitation efforts.
Address individual and family psychodynamic issues that interfere with acceptance of the illness and participation in rehabilitative treatment.
Engage professional colleagues and treatment systems that can facilitate treatment for patients with chronic mental illness.

Dr. Transome, too, is confronted with an acute exacerbation of a chronic psychotic disorder. He must face the pressures of the attitudes of the ward staff and the patient's family—reflections of the demoralization that often infects those persons responsible for the care of individuals with chronic, intractable illness. Once Dr. Transome completes the task of controlling his patient's acute psychotic episode, he will confront the more difficult job of providing an extended plan of management that might stimulate both the patient's medication compliance and his hope for a better life. At the same time, Dr. Transome needs to combat the family's "burnout" and to alleviate their despair and hopelessness.

Similarly, Dr. Lyon, subjected to the erratic and provocative behavior of Ms. Debarry and the resistant attitude of her mother, experiences in the outpatient clinic a challenge similar to Dr. Holt's in the emergency room. Like Dr. Holt and Dr. Transome, Dr. Lyon must first stabilize a crisis and then devise a long-range treatment plan that anticipates and tries to prevent other similar crises as therapy progresses.

Before going on to specific suggestions regarding the assessment and treatment of each of these three patients, we will describe the basic conceptual framework that we recommend for assessing and treating chronically mentally ill individuals.

The Strategy of Treatment

To provide appropriate and effective treatment for individuals with chronic mental illness, the resident needs to develop a clear conceptual framework that defines both the therapeutic task and the therapeutic process. This framework includes three basic elements:

1. **The biological roots.** An appreciation of the biological underpinnings of major mental illness that underlie both the *vulnerability* to such illness and the *chronicity* of the consequent disability.
2. **The psychosocial component.** Incorporation of the psychodynamic, social, familial, and environmental factors that provide the basis for a thorough understanding of the *person* who has the disorder, the *family* that is affected by it, and the *system* of services that is designed to help them.
3. **The long-term rehabilitation process.** A process to engender hope in patient, family, and therapist throughout the long course of the illness so that as patients and families confront the painful reality of chronic and almost incurable mental illness, they remain aware of the possibility for *progress* and *recovery,* even for those patients suffering from the most profound and persistent disorders.

The Biological Roots of Mental Illness: The Disease Model

Major mental illness has its roots in biological processes. Although this may be obvious in the abstract, it is often not fully understood by either patients or clinicians. Schizophrenia and the affective psychoses are biological in the sense that biological vulnerability is a necessary condition for the development of the disorders. Psychological, familial, social, and environmental variables help to determine the onset and the idiosyncratic character of the symptoms, and to influence their clinical course, but the predisposing biological vulnerability is the essential variable for the development of the illness.

Characteristics of chronic mental illness that may have a biological basis and that are important to emphasize because of their crucial impact on treatment include

1. **Chronicity.** Although not all patients with schizophrenia and affective psychosis develop a chronic course, the majority do. Chronicity implies that the illness—or the risk of relapse—persists, to some degree, for a long time—often for the patient's entire life.
2. **Potential for deterioration.** While people with schizophrenia and affective psychosis can be treated successfully and can make progress, they may deteriorate if the disease is untreated, or if they are repeatedly noncompliant.
3. **Denial.** Denial is a common characteristic of chronic mental illnesses that may be related, at least in part, to the cognitive deficits associated with the psychotic process. The chronically psychotic patient who cannot accurately perceive the severity of his or her illness is likely not to comply with treatment, and consequently to have a poor outcome.
4. **Disability.** Even when these illnesses are stabilized with medication, significant disability often remains. This disability may be *primary,* resulting from continuation of symptoms or ongoing deficits in cognitive processing due to the illness; *secondary,* due to lack of motivation or demoralization resulting from persistent symptoms; and/or *tertiary,* due to social rejection or stigma as a consequence of exhibiting illness-related behavior. All three types of disability are a direct result of the biological disorder and must be addressed for treatment to proceed.

The disease model, with its concept of biological vulnerability, has several important implications for treatment tactics, as outlined in Table 1–2. The first two steps are to make an accurate diagnosis and a thorough assessment of the severity of the acute illness—both crucial prerequisites for treatment. The third and most urgent step is to stabilize the symptoms through pharmacological and other physical treatments. The fourth step, once the acute symptoms are stabilized, is to assess the patient's symptomatology, social skills, and vocational functioning at *baseline.* Meanwhile, it is important to attempt to relieve the patient and family of blame for *causing* the biological illness, and at the same time to mobilize the patient and family as allies in managing the illness. If blame and associated feelings of failure and guilt can be alleviated, the doctor, patient, and family can more easily become collaborators in the management of the illness and in the process of rehabilitation.

Table 1–2. Tactics of management of chronically mentally ill patients

Disease model: treating the biological illness

1. Make an accurate diagnosis.
2. Assess severity of acute illness.
3. Stabilize symptoms pharmacologically.
4. Assess *baseline* functioning.
5. Relieve patient and family of responsibility for causing the illness.
6. Mobilize patient and family as allies in managing the illness.

Psychosocial component: treating the person

1. Perform multidimensional, longitudinal assessment.
2. Educate patient and family to overcome denial.
3. Implement a plan to prevent treatment noncompliance.
4. Help patient and family develop new coping skills.

Long-term program of rehabilitation and recovery

1. Maintain long-term stabilization and treatment compliance.
2. Define attainable "next step" goals and objectives.
3. Develop long-term treatment plan to attain these goals.
4. Address ongoing feelings of impatience and frustration to maintain the proper pace of progress.
5. Help patient and family to maximize self-acceptance, autonomy, and satisfaction with life despite persistence of the illness.

The Psychosocial Component: Treating the Person, Not Just the Disease

Although recognizing the biological factors in mental illness is essential for proper treatment, it is equally important for the physician to recognize and explore the psychological, familial, social, and environmental aspects of the chronic disorder. Effective treatment is based on an integrated view of the patient as a person and an understanding of the multiple forces that determine the course of the patient's whole life as a person with a mental illness. The same integrated view requires an empathic understanding of family members as well. Because patient, family, and clinician are contending with an incurable disease, the focus of treatment shifts from "curing" illness to helping the persons who suffer from the illness—that is, helping them to understand, accept, and adapt to the illness. The clinician can begin by exploring individual and family feelings about the illness and its impact, and can then help the family work through resistances to accepting the limitations imposed by the illness.

The emergence of symptoms of major mental illness is an overwhelmingly stressful occurrence for both patient and family, and their lives are always radically changed. The resident's empathic recognition of the impact of this change facilitates patient and family involvement in adaptation and rehabilitation, which requires examination of individual and family styles of behavior that increase the liability to relapse and to impede progress.

The specific psychosocial management tactics, outlined in Table 1–2, are discussed in more detail below.

1. **Multidimensional, longitudinal assessment.** In any medical setting, residents first establish rapport with their patients and then collect the data necessary to arrive at a specific diagnosis. In the case of patients with *chronic* illness, medical *or* psychiatric, the diagnosis is only a beginning. Assessment must go beyond the label to include a description of the longitudinal course and the prognosis of the illness, its idiosyncracies in the patient under observation, the extent of its concomitant disabilities, and its physical, psychological, familial, and social impact.

   Thus, on the inpatient ward, Dr. Transome will not only prescribe and adjust the patient's medication, but also explore the impact of the illness on the lives of Mr. Jermyn and his family, and use this information to develop a comprehensive longitudinal multidimensional assessment and treatment plan.
2. **Education to overcome denial.** All patients and families wish that the illness did not exist—a wish that engenders the denial and minimization that so often blocks therapeutic efforts. The resident needs patience to help chronically mentally ill persons and their family members to work through their denial and to come to terms with the fact that they are dealing with a chronic condition that requires long and continuous treatment. The resident fosters acceptance by teaching the patient and the family about the nature of the illness and the treatments, biological and psychological, that are required to combat it. Even those persons who seem to understand and accept the illness need repeated explanations, particularly as the illness drags on and despair and denial threaten to recur in the face of lengthening chronicity and persistent disability.
3. **Prevention of noncompliance.** Denial impairs patients' ability to comply with treatment, especially in the early stages. Patients with any chronic illness can feel so much better as treatment takes effect

that they begin to believe they no longer require medication. Diabetic patients, for example, once the acute symptoms are under control, may stop taking their insulin or give up their diets. In the same way, mentally ill patients, like Mr. Jermyn, may discontinue medication once they are stabilized.

In addition to denial, such issues as annoying side effects, a change in therapist, concomitant substance abuse, or underlying despair and hopelessness may contribute to noncompliance. Dr. Transome needs to explore these and other possibilities with Mr. Jermyn and his family to prevent or moderate future relapses.

4. **The acquisition of coping skills.** Acceptance of the illness and education about its nature are preludes to the acquisition of new skills for coping with being chronically ill. These may include coping with chronic psychotic symptoms; bearing feelings of hopelessness, frustration, anxiety, and despair; developing flexibility in responding to changing treatment needs during different phases of the illness and convalescence; recognizing and responding to the prodromal signs of relapse; dealing with the intricacies of the mental health system; learning to cope with or overcome chronic disabilities; and many others.

Developing new skills facilitates the maintenance of stability, which in turn allows more new skills to be developed. Slowly, over time, the patient and family can learn to accept the illness and its treatment more calmly and to acknowledge the limitations and disabilities that the illness imposes with a greater sense of peace of mind. This calmness promotes maximum functioning within those limitations and stimulates further emotional and rehabilitative growth.

Ms. DeBarry, for example, requires skillful management from Dr. Lyon as she unconsciously foments crisis after crisis in a desperate attempt to obtain from others the strength and control she lacks. As a stable therapeutic relationship with Dr. Lyon slowly develops, Ms. DeBarry can acquire the ability to moderate her feelings and to ask for help more appropriately. This will in turn help her to feel more in control of her life, as well as her illness, and will lay the groundwork for further therapeutic progress.

A Realistic Long-Term Program of Rehabilitation and Recovery

Maintaining hope in the face of a chronic, incurable illness often seems like an impossible paradox. Patients, families, and clinicians easily succumb to the despairing mind-set that defines continuing symptoms and persistent disability as indications of a hopeless prognosis.

As we view it, however, the *successful* outcome is defined by acceptance, relative peace of mind, and progress to the "next step," rather than by the total elimination of symptoms or the attainment of such normative goals as independent living or competitive employment. Moreover, increased acceptance of persistent symptoms can actually lead to gradual symptom reduction and increased comfort, with slow progress to the "next step." This process of acceptance can lead to more progress than can pressure to make great leaps forward (see Table 1–2).

Although the progress of "treatment" in chronic mental illness can sometimes proceed over 20 to 30 years—a process that is frustratingly slow for patients, families, and residents alike—residents can learn to accomplish and appreciate substantial gains even within 1 to 2 years of treatment. For example, Dr. Holt can develop a therapeutic relationship with Ms. Hogarth and her mother that will increase acceptance of the disease and promote improved coping skills in order to prevent recurrent visits to the emergency room and to maintain stability in the workshop. Dr. Transome can encourage Mr. Jermyn and his parents to develop a strategy for requiring Mr. Jermyn to accept intramuscularly administered medication as a condition for living at home. Dr. Lyon can engage Ms. DeBarry in a stabilizing treatment relationship that could lead to a reduction in crisis behavior and might evolve into meaningful long-term psychotherapy, as noted above. Attainment of these so-called "limited" goals can engender a sense of pride, accomplishment, and satisfaction and can lead to further and more rewarding long-term involvement with patients and their families.

2

Engagement With and Assessment of Chronically Mentally Ill Patients

Mary Hogarth (continued from p. 3)

In the emergency room, after Mary Hogarth has accepted the can of ginger ale and has somewhat calmed down, Dr. Holt feels more assured of her own and the patient's safety. She begins to try to persuade Ms. Hogarth to accept voluntary admission, saying, "I'm Dr. Holt, Ms. Hogarth, and I've been talking with your mother. She tells me that some things at work have been upsetting you. Could you tell me something about them?"

Mrs. Hogarth launches into an obviously delusional account of murders and plots. Dr. Holt listens attentively, meanwhile trying to figure out how to get Mary to go peacefully to the ward. It occurs to Dr. Holt that if she were in Ms. Hogarth's shoes and were convinced that her delusions were true, she too would be terrified. So, at a break in the story, she says, "It must be upsetting and frightening to feel that all these things are going on and nobody but you seems to be aware of them. You must feel so alone."

This empathic comment brings about an abrupt change in Ms. Hogarth's feelings, from anger to tears. This change, although surprising Dr. Holt, makes it possible for her gently to encourage Ms. Hogarth to accept help in dealing with her frightening experiences by admitting herself to the hospital: "In the hospital, you will be kept safe, so no one will hurt you, and there will be staff round the clock to talk to you and help you to feel more calm. Plus, we can adjust your medication so that it works better."

When Ms. Hogarth's mother sees that Dr. Holt has gained her daughter's trust, she is more willing to allow hospitalization. Her willingness is reinforced by Dr. Holt's explanation that adjustment of

Mary's medication would be more safely accomplished in a hospital setting, where careful observation of side effects can occur. Dr. Holt then goes up to the ward with Ms. Hogarth and her mother, explains the entrance procedures, tells them that another resident, Dr. Dickens, would be Mary's doctor while she is on the ward, and writes initial medication orders.

As Dr. Holt leaves the ward, she thinks to herself that she has actually done a pretty good job. Not only has she overcome her apprehension, but she has succeeded in engaging a frightening patient. In fact, somewhat to her surprise, Dr. Holt realizes that she feels sorry that the rotation of assignments will not allow her to be Mary's ward doctor.

Building Rapport With Chronically Mentally Ill Patients

Dr. Holt's experience with Ms. Hogarth illustrates how rapport can be established by engaging the patient in empathic communication in a context that ensures the safety of both the patient and the clinician. Ideally, rapport is established before the assessment. During a psychiatric crisis, however, this ideal must often be sacrificed and rapport must be established during, rather than before, the assessment. As we saw in Chapter 1, Drs. Holt, Transome, and Lyon had little time to develop rapport before they had to begin their diagnostic assessment, and they did not have much time to develop a specific diagnosis before having to initiate preliminary treatment.

Although the same pressure to bypass normal procedures occurs in medical crises, the patients in such cases are usually more passively accepting of what is done for them; the clues to what is wrong are more likely to be in physical or laboratory data than in psychological data; and the course is ordinarily not quite as unpredictable. Consequently, rapport, while always desirable, is not as immediately essential for initiating the treatment of the medical patient in crisis as it is for initiating the crisis treatment of the chronically mentally ill patient.

Safety, empathy, and *communication* are the key elements in developing rapport and engaging the patient. In the following sections, we will discuss specific approaches for addressing these issues as the resident engages the individual patient in a treatment relationship.

Addressing Issues of Safety

A major barrier to developing rapport with the chronically mentally ill patient is the resident's concern both about his or her own safety and about the patient's safety. In the emergency room, Mary Hogarth looked as if she were ready "to strike out at any moment"; on the inpatient unit, Mr. Jermyn's posture was often "threatening"; and in the outpatient clinic, Ms. DeBarry spoke of suicide. Because the reasons for each patient's anger and possible violent or suicidal behavior were obscure, accurate prediction was impossible; as long as the resident felt uncertain about whether the patients were safe or dangerous, it was difficult to build rapport. Residents, therefore, need to create first of all a safe context in which empathic communication can occur before further assessment can begin.

Preventing Violence

The prevention of violence starts in the emergency room, where the risks of violence are greatest. Before meeting a new patient, the resident can inquire of staff, family, friends, or police officers if there is a history of violent behavior and under what circumstances the patient came to the hospital. With patients who behave violently prior to admission, who appear to be intoxicated and unpredictable, and who are brought in against their will, the resident may decide to conduct the interview in the presence of security personnel; at the least, security staff should be readily available. Residents also can ensure the possibility of a rapid retreat by not permitting threatening or angry patients to get between them and the door.

Usually the presence of security guards or police as a show of strength allows the resident to take control of the situation. Occasionally, however, control of the patient may require physical and/or chemical restraint. Residents often fear that such measures will inhibit rapport, and thus they may wait too long to institute them in hopes of calming the patient verbally. However, some patients may remain assaultive and frightening no matter how much and what kind of reassurance they receive. In such cases, the resident must trust his or her perceptions and not be ashamed of any apprehensive feelings. It is much better to take precautions—even if in retrospect they were unnecessary—than to risk injury to patient and staff by trying to be heroic. The following case illustrates this issue:

> Dr. Stuart, a psychiatric resident, first meets Ms. Nickles, a 25-year-old woman with a 5-year history of schizophrenia with intermittent hospitalization, when her mother brings her to the mental health clinic because Ms. Nickles has suffered a relapse. Unable to sit still, Ms. Nickles speaks rapidly in a grandiose manner, talking vaguely about being persecuted by the Mafia.

After talking with her for a few minutes about her symptoms, Dr. Stuart, realizing that the patient urgently needs hospital care, leaves the room to call the ambulance. When he returns, he tentatively broaches the idea of hospitalization, but Ms. Nickles strongly objects and does not want to hear about it. Dr. Stuart then turns to her mother to discuss how he can get the patient to agree to a voluntary admission. The patient, apparently guessing his intention, becomes panicky and runs out of the room onto a porch above the street. When Dr. Stuart follows her, hoping to calm her until the ambulance arrives, he finds her holding a flower pot over her head. He is not sure whether she would jump from the porch to the street or try to smash his head with the pot. Fortunately, the ambulance arrives just then, and two experienced attendants take the pot away from her and drive her to the hospital.

This case illustrates how important it is to establish rapport, if the patient's voluntary cooperation is required, and to provide control, if the patient is likely to resist. The resident stated later that he had learned from the experience the risks both of prematurely discussing voluntary hospitalization with patients and of being indecisive instead of taking control. Ms. Nickles' behavior was alarming enough to indicate that additional assistance was needed, and security personnel should have been notified to be ready for intervention *before* the resident even mentioned hospitalization.

Some of the techniques residents can use to prevent violence (see Table 2–1) are discussed below.

Maintaining adequate distance. Although it is important to establish a trusting relationship with potentially violent patients, building rapport does not mean trying too hard to make patients admire and like us. With potentially out-of-control patients, especially those with schizophrenia, too much emotional intensity and physical closeness may be frightening and can actually increase the risk of violence. Such patients, therefore, need a calm, low-key approach that is sensitive to maintaining

Table 2–1. Some techniques for the prevention of violence in potentially violent patients

Maintain adequate physical and emotional distance.
Set clear limits rather than placate the patient.
Reduce the level of stimulation.
Ensure the presence of adequate security.
Use physical and chemical restraints without hesitation when necessary.
Be prepared to implement involuntary commitment.

adequate physical distance. Assessing how much distance is "adequate" requires careful observation of the patient as the resident slowly approaches, being prepared to back off if the patient appears to become more anxious.

Setting clear limits. Setting appropriate—but not rigid or punitive—limits and boundaries shows the out-of-control patient that the clinician cares and is trying to prevent harm. Thus, in the long run, appropriate limit setting facilitates rather than inhibits the development of rapport. By contrast, responding to each expressed wish to such patients may increase their anxiety and demandingness by giving the impression that the resident is scared to take control.

Reducing overstimulation. Acutely decompensated psychotic patients are often hyperalert and exquisitely sensitive to the level of stimulation in their environment. Whenever possible, with such patients it is best to decrease the level of stimulation by placing the patients in a quiet area, under observation but with minimal interaction, and to converse with them calmly and slowly.

Ensuring adequate security. Before initiating any intervention or interaction that might agitate the patient, the resident must be certain that adequate security is present to prevent the patient from attacking or bolting. *Setting limits* on a demanding patient is best carried out by having security personnel present to forestall an explosion by the patient once the limit is imposed.

Using restraints. Establishing good rapport and setting the stage for a therapeutic relationship are not inconsistent with physical restraint of the agitated and potentially destructive patient. If talking to such patients in a calm way and persuading them to accept medication are not successful, the resident may have to resort to physical restraints. Such a last-resort decision is always hard on both patient and physician. However, if restraints are humanely handled, and if the patients are released from restraints as soon as they have gained some self-control, they later may express their appreciation for the staff's having protected them and others from themselves.

Involuntary commitment. Many residents are reluctant to initiate involuntary commitment because of concerns about alienating the patient or infringing his or her rights. Yet in most instances the courage to commit is a caring, protective act in which the patient's safety is ensured and the possibility of a relationship created. In the process of commitment, it is helpful for the resident to state clearly his or her intent, even in the face of the patient's rage, as by saying:

> Your behavior is out of control and dangerous. In order to ensure your safety and keep you from causing harm, we must hospitalize you. Because you cannot agree to this voluntarily right now, emergency commitment will be necessary. I know this is frightening, but we will make every effort to keep you as safe and as calm as possible. I will be happy to discuss this further with you when you are feeling better.

The potentially assaultive patient is usually terrified. Imagine how frightening it must be to lose your ability to understand the surrounding world and to be convinced that you are the target of strong and harmful influences, or that you are about to be cruelly punished by shadowy and disguised persecutors. In response to the perceived inner terror and in an effort to defend themselves against imaginary enemies, some patients assume threatening poses and frighten other people. When they sense the fear they have created in others, they become even more frightened of counterattack.

Before such patients can be expected to calm down and cooperate in an interview, they need to be tranquilized—not only by pharmacological means but also by the soothing presence of a reassuring, empathic person. It is hard to be empathic, however, if you are preoccupied with your own fear. Furthermore, your fear actually heightens the risk of assault by agitated patients. The resident can learn to project a calm, measured, confident approach, keeping in mind that the patient is more terrified of him or her than the reverse, as is seen in the following example:

> John Thompson, a 25-year-old man with a long-standing diagnosis of paranoid schizophrenia, has had several episodes of violent behavior on the ward. These episodes have usually occurred in the evenings and on weekends when Dr. Green, the resident, is away. Dr. Green has tried, without success, to identify the precipitants of these episodes.
>
> One morning, the night nurse calls Dr. Green at 6:30 A.M. The patient has dismantled his bed and retreated to a corner of his room, threatening to club with a bedpost anyone who approaches him. When Dr. Green arrives, he finds two frightened male attendants outside the patient's door and the night nurse hovering in the background. All of them are watching the patient apprehensively and obviously looking for guidance to the resident, who himself is uncertain how to deal with this emergency.
>
> Fortunately, the chief nurse just then arrives on duty. Half the size of the patient, she quickly sizes up the situation, pushes the attendants aside, and walks into the room. "John," she says in a calm and reassur-

> ing voice, "I am here now and no one's going to hurt you. You can tell me what's frightening you. Meanwhile, please give me the bedpost, and I'll take care of it." The patient hands her the bedpost, sits down, and tells her that the voices have been threatening him. The nurse patiently explains that the voices are part of his illness, and asks him whether something has upset him to aggravate his symptoms.
>
> Later, the chief tells Dr. Green, "I wouldn't have gone in there if I didn't know that Mr. Thompson trusted me. I never take chances with violent patients unless I know them and I can convey to them that I am there to help and not to hurt them."

Familiarity breeds trust; the chief nurse provides a reassuring continuity on the ward in contrast to that provided by the more transient and less experienced night and weekend staff.

Frightened, out-of-control patients often need to be reassured that "thinking" and "feeling" differ from "acting," a distinction that some patients have trouble accepting. These patients need to know that if they talk about their angry feelings, they may in fact gain control over them. In the following case, a resident's calm, empathic exploration of a patient's hostile impulses successfully reduced the patient's urgency to act on them:

> The charge nurse notices that Mr. Weller, a 23-year-old college student who usually keeps quietly to himself, has become agitated. Mr. Weller had been admitted a week earlier after he had repeatedly called police to complain that his neighbors were spying on him and trying to find out about his sex life. In the last hour he had begun to pace furiously in the day room, occasionally muttering to himself.
>
> The nurse calls Dr. Stovall, who gently asks the patient if he feels like talking. Seemingly relieved, the patient agrees. [If the patient had become *more* agitated, Dr. Stovall might then have contacted security personnel to be present.] The patient says that he is worried that he might be a homosexual. Another young man had recently been admitted to the ward, and the patient believes that the patients and nurses are watching to see whether he will make a pass at the new patient. As he becomes more upset, he begins to suspect that fellow patients are referring to him as "queer." He has been fighting off thoughts of attacking the other young man and "getting rid of him" because he blames him for his distress.
>
> Dr. Stovall commends Mr. Weller for his frankness, reassures him (without arguing) that he is not being referred to as a "queer," and suggests that they continue to explore his concern about his sexual orientation. At the same time he also suggests an increase in the medication that would help the patient to regain his self-control. The patient appears to be much calmer after the interview.

In summary, the resident can ensure safety with even the most violent patient by establishing an atmosphere of clear limits and calm control. Ensuring safety may range from simply ensuring the presence and availability of security personnel to use of physical restraint and involuntary commitment. Only when the resident feels reasonably safe can he or she begin calmly to establish empathic contact, which in turn can lead the patient to feel safer and thus can reduce the need for external limits and controls. Even if the resident is not feeling completely calm, it helps for him or her to try to appear calm. The most important lesson is that the resident must trust his or her own feelings and not try to be heroic by taking unnecessary risks.

A similar set of principles determines measures for ensuring safety with patients who are suicidal.

Preventing Self-Injury

Just as with potentially violent patients, residents must be sure, in order to create a safe climate for establishing rapport, that potentially suicidal patients are protected from harming themselves. Because suicidal patients are typically experiencing considerable distress, an empathic approach is usually sufficient to persuade them to accept treatment. Whether to hospitalize an ambulatory patient or refer him or her for intensive outpatient crisis intervention depends on the clinician's assessment of the patient's ability to contract reliably for safety—that is, to agree and to live up to the agreement to see the clinician or to check in at the emergency room before doing anything self-destructive. The decision also depends on the patient's responsiveness to the initial contact and the availability of collateral supports, such as the family.

If a patient expresses suicidal intent or exhibits suicidal behavior, as by overdosing, and then refuses or resists help, the resident must assume that the patient is not safe and must take steps to contain the patient until safety is established. These steps should include the following:

1. Maintaining constant security observation of any suicidal patient until an initial assessment has been completed and the patient is considered able to manage with less supervision.
2. Explaining to patient and family that the patient cannot be released until the resident is satisfied either that enough safeguards are available to keep the patient safe or that the patient is sufficiently improved to be able to reliably guarantee his or her own safety.
3. Being prepared to initiate involuntary hospitalization if safety cannot otherwise be ensured; in such circumstances patients will often consent to engage in treatment in order to avoid being committed.

Suicidal patients, as well as violent patients, tend to respond to a resident's sense of calm control combined with an empathic, caring approach. At the same time, the resident will learn to trust his or her own subjective feelings about a patient's safety or reliability, and will use these feelings as a guide. Once a patient expresses suicidal intent, the burden is on the patient to demonstrate that he or she is safe.

Although the approach outlined above is relatively easy to implement with most suicidal patients, patients who are also chronically mentally ill may present particular difficulties for the beginning resident. For example, some patients' suicidal communications may be so bizarre and/or indirect that the resident is left wondering whether to take these communications seriously. These patients may be so disorganized, delusional, confused, or impulsive that the resident may not believe that in each case the patient can make a reliable contract.

The following example illustrates how one such situation was handled:

Mr. Smythe, a 42-year-old patient with chronic schizophrenia, wanders into the emergency room one evening complaining that he feels that he is going to die. After presenting a bizarre litany of medical symptoms, he is found to be medically clear and is referred to Dr. Johnson, the psychiatric resident on call:

DR. JOHNSON: What seems to be the problem?

MR. SMYTHE: I'm going to die.

DR. J.: When?

MR. S.: Probably tonight.

DR. J.: How do you know?

MR. S.: God has been talking to me. He gave me a sign—a pain in my heart. He wants me to save mankind and be resurrected, like Jesus Christ.

DR. J.: How will this happen?

MR. S.: I'm not sure. God will let me know what to do.

DR. J.: Do you mean—to kill yourself?

MR. S.: No, of course not. God will do it.

DR. J.: Are you upset about this?

MR. S.: No, I trust in Him. Do you believe in God?

DR. J.: Yes, I do. But I'm curious about something. If you felt O.K. about this, why did you come here tonight?

MR. S.: I'm not sure. I think God told me that I should die in a hospital, but now I'm not sure. Maybe I should just go home. [*Starts to leave.*]

DR. J. [*feeling anxious, but grateful that he had asked security to wait outside in case the patient tried to bolt*]: I don't think that's a good idea. I think there must have been a very important reason why you heard God directing you to come here tonight, and I think you need to stay and find out what it was. We'll make sure you are safe.

MR. S.: Well, maybe. I guess, though, that I'll have to go wherever God sends me.

Although Dr. Johnson cannot discover the patient's actual suicidal intentions, the patient reveals enough about the psychotic process to make Dr. Johnson very concerned. Dr. Johnson also recognizes that the patient is ambivalent about dying, which is why "God" directed him to the hospital. By carefully allying with the patient's world view—without actually agreeing with the delusion—Dr. Johnson can persuade Mr. Smythe to accept help. If Mr. Smythe refuses and insists on leaving, Dr. Johnson will have to restrain him:

MR. S.: No. I really must be going.

DR. J.: I'm sorry, but I'm concerned for your safety, and I cannot let you leave until I'm sure that you won't die.

MR. S.: But God wants me to die.

DR. J.: I know that's how you see it, but you may be mistaken, and I need to keep you safe to make sure you don't die by mistake.

Dr. Johnson has security stay with the patient while he contacts family, friends, caregivers, and clinicians who know Mr. Smythe for more information. If he is not reassured that Mr. Smythe will be safe, he will arrange for involuntary hospitalization.

Many chronically mentally ill individuals have difficulty engaging in outpatient treatment or in maintaining a treatment alliance. Some of these patients, like Ms. DeBarry (see Chapter 1, pp. 6–8), may also exhibit self-injurious or provocative behavior that legitimately arouses concern for their safety. Such behaviors include using medications inappropriately, as by skipping doses, overdosing, or both; cutting, burning, or otherwise injuring themselves; expressing suicidal ideas and then missing appointments or refusing to discuss the ideas; and breaking treatment contracts and abusing substances in association with self-destructive ideas (see Chapter 10). As with the violent patient, gently setting limits can be reassuring to the out-of-control self-destructive patient and can facilitate, rather than inhibit, the development of rapport, even if involuntary hospitalization is required:

Ms. Sawyer, a disorganized schizophrenic woman with a history of impulsive overdoses while on passes, was released from the state hospital to the care of her parents and the family psychiatrist. A contract was established as a condition of her release that any selfdestructive behavior would result in immediate rehospitalization for at least a week. (The patient could also voluntarily request hospitalization for periods of respite if she wished.)

Approximately 3 months after discharge, the patient takes a small overdose after an argument with her mother. The contract is enforced, and no further overdoses occur. The patient tells her psychiatrist that she feels he must really care, because he tries so hard to protect her.

In summary, the prevention of self-injury in chronically mentally ill patients requires application of the same basic principles as for other patients, but with special attention to the indirect nature of much of the patients' communication and to their capacity for impulsivity and unpredictability. In all instances, the resident's calm, empathic, but firm control helps to support these patients' ability to remain safe.

Using Empathy to Establish Rapport

A resident's first clinical contact with a chronically mentally ill patient may not be his or her first experience with such a patient. Before their psychiatric residencies began, Drs. Holt, Transome, and Lyon (see Chapter 1) all had had encounters with psychiatric patients, but primarily as medical students in the role of observers. Because they were not then in charge of their patients' care, they could maintain more psychological distance than they can now as resident physicians who are responsible for their patients' treatment.

As participants, residents at first may find it easier to think about patients in terms of the observable, measurable diagnostic criteria in DSM-III-R, and more difficult to consider such phenomena as feelings, thoughts, fantasies, and dreams as being equally significant. Yet it is the awareness of these subjective data that sets the stage for empathy, and empathy is the key to working with patients with chronic mental illness.

Empathy is not always easy to develop or maintain with chronically mentally ill patients for several reasons:

1. Disorganized or bizarre behavior may evoke patronizing, distancing, or rejecting responses.
2. Psychosis is usually not part of the resident's own experience and is unfamiliar and frightening.
3. The lack of control inherent in the patient's experience may be threatening to the resident, who is trying to maintain a sense of order and control in his or her own training.

4. Despair, disability, and chronicity may be difficult to accept and experience for a successful, hopeful, achievement-oriented resident.
5. Patients may be regarded as childlike, dependent, or incomplete and somehow less than fully real or human.
6. Many patients are negligent about grooming, bathing, and hygiene, and may exhibit repugnant behaviors or unpleasant body odor.
7. Many chronic patients (such as Ms. Hogarth, Mr. Jermyn, and Ms. DeBarry) are already well-known and have tainted reputations, thus negatively influencing the resident even before the first meeting.

To overcome these problems, residents can observe the following simple guidelines (summarized in Table 2–2):

1. As you imagine yourself in the patient's predicament, ask yourself: How would I feel if I heard voices no one else heard? How would I feel if I were given a Prolixin shot against my will?
2. Think of patients as persons with bizarre illnesses rather than as bizarre persons; this perspective will help to make their experience more accessible.
3. Listen to the patient's affective tone and resist premature intervention. The more carefully you listen to affective tone as well as to content, and the more you resist the urge to intervene prematurely, the more likely you are to be able to respond empathically to the feelings behind the patient's speech.
4. Respond empathically to the patient's feelings of inadequacy, shame, despair, and incapacity, even when these feelings are not directly expressed.
5. Respect the patient's autonomy and humanity. Because chronically mentally ill patients are extremely sensitive to condescension and humiliation, one might say in introducing oneself: "Ms. Hogarth, I'm Dr. Holt. Would you prefer that I call you Ms. Hogarth or Mary?"

Table 2–2. Guidelines for building empathy with chronic patients

Imagine yourself with a chronic illness.
Think of the patient as a normal person with a terrible illness.
Listen to affective tone as well as content.
Focus on feelings of defectiveness, shame, despair, and incapacity.
Treat the patient with respect.
View all behaviors as meaningful cues to understanding.
Communicate empathy clearly.

6. Remind yourself that all behaviors and symptoms have meaning and are clues to understanding the patient as a person. Even the most repugnant appearance can be seen as a sad indication of the patient's level of dysfunction and despair.
7. Communicate your empathic understanding as much as possible in clear, simple language, as by saying, "It must be scary to hear voices and not be able to get rid of them," or "It can be depressing to be sick and unable to work."

Overcoming Barriers to Communication

When assessing a chronically mentally ill patient, even beginning the process of communication can be difficult. Many chronic patients, like Ms. Hogarth (the patient seen by Dr. Holt in the emergency room [Chapter 1, pp. 1–3]), will talk only about their symptoms and will not talk about what has happened. In Ms. Hogarth's case, Dr. Holt, under pressure to get enough data together to make a decision about Ms. Hogarth's disposition, might have been tempted to try to persuade her to divulge the details of the episode that led to the trip to the emergency room by saying, for example, "I'm a physician, and it's perfectly safe to [or, you have to] tell me what happened."

From Dr. Holt's point of view, it was indeed perfectly safe to talk with the patient, but from Ms. Hogarth's point of view, it would have been just the opposite. Even if the patient had not provided clues to her view of the world by her delusional account of murders and plots, Dr. Holt could assume that, along with most other chronically mentally ill patients, Ms. Hogarth's trust in others, especially others in authority, had been severely impaired. So for Ms. Hogarth it was not safe at that time to talk about what had happened to her, and it could have been desperately important for her to resist coercion. Dr. Holt had to wait for the details until rapport had been established, unless she found such information out from the staff at work.

Nonverbal communication is also important, particularly when its message contradicts the patient's words:

DR. HOLT: You don't have to be afraid; I am only trying to help you.

MS. HOGARTH: I'm not afraid.

If the patient gives this response while seated comfortably in a chair, hands relaxed and face in repose, it is probably safe to take the patient's words at face value. But if the patient is cringing in the corner of the chair, fists clenched and eyes darting back and forth, "I'm not afraid" may mean "I am afraid, but too afraid of you to say anything but what you expect me to say."

Actually, although most doctors—and most people—evaluate others' verbal communication in the nonverbal context, they are less likely to evaluate their own nonverbal behavior. Cordial, welcoming expressions and gestures facilitate rapport; angry or contemptuous body language does just the opposite. At one time, offering the patient a cigarette contributed to breaking the ice; these days cigarettes are taboo, but an offer to get the patient a soda, as in Mary Hogarth's case (see p. 3), can have the same effect.

Mary Hogarth (continued from p. 18)

By the time Dr. Lincoln, the resident responsible for Ms. Hogarth's assessment, sees Ms. Hogarth, the patient has been reassured by Dr. Holt's empathic manner and by a night in the protected atmosphere of the ward. After describing her symptoms and finding that Dr. Lincoln listens and does not argue with her about them, she may be ready to talk about the circumstances of their onset. On the other hand, she may still be hesitant to discuss them; if so, Dr. Lincoln may have to use an unthreatening approach such as, "I can see that you're upset, and I'd like to help you, but to do so, I'll have to know more about how things that concern you got started."

The patient may respond as the doctor wants her to if she is not too distrustful, or else she may still perceive the doctor's encouragement as a trap to force her to talk when she is afraid to do so.

As in most medical and psychiatric cases, both Dr. Holt and Dr. Lincoln find that relating to Ms. Hogarth where she is—ruminating about murders—rather than where they would like her to be—telling them about precipitants—is the best way to facilitate communication. What each resident does is simply to empathize with her—to let her know that someone is trying to understand her. Understanding her is not the same as agreeing with her; the doctors do not acknowledge that murders have in fact occurred, only that they understand how upsetting it is for the patient to believe that murders have occurred. Trying to argue patients out of their delusions is almost always futile; the alternative is to walk the tightrope between arguing and agreeing, acknowledging that while you recognize that the perceptions are real to the patient, you do not share them:

PATIENT: How can you help me if you don't believe what I tell you?

DOCTOR: It isn't that I don't believe that these (delusions, etc.) are real to you; it's that I don't have the same perception of them that you have.

To carry this process a step further, you might ask how others react to the patient's hallucinations or delusions. If the patient says that others do not share them and, in fact, try to argue with the patient, you might empathically comment on how frustrating that must be, and suggest that the patient talk about them only with you, because you understand how upsetting these delusions are, even if you view them differently. In this way, an alliance can be formed that permits the patient to trust you enough to give more information and at the same time reduces the extent to which others become alienated.

Communication presents special problems when patients are mute; when their communications are incomprehensible or irrelevant; when patients are delusional about the doctor; or when they are paranoid.

When the patient is mute. Some patients are completely mute, and others are too frightened, angry, suspicious, or depressed to talk beyond a few monosyllables. Such patients are frustrating, especially if they talk freely to other patients, to family members, or to the nursing staff. Expressing frustration about this lack of cooperation directly to the patient, however, is not likely to result in better rapport. More promising routes to communication are consistent efforts to gain patients' trust by showing interest in and addressing their immediate needs, reacting with patience and equanimity, demonstrating empathy, and exploring possible meanings of the resistance to talking. The meaning might be explored by a straightforward question such as the following: "I wonder if you could tell me what frightens you so much about sharing thoughts with me?" Such an approach shifts the focus from the symptoms themselves to the patient's resistance to talking about the symptoms.

If a patient remains uncommunicative, other sources—family, friends, police officers, or whoever brought the patient to the hospital—can provide information. Meanwhile, a foundation for later communication may be laid by an approach such as "I suspect that there are some things you would like to tell me, but that you are somehow scared to say. I'd like to be able to help you, so if there's any way, by words or gestures or whatever, that you can let me know how I can help, please do so—either now or later."

A common reason for patients to fear talking is the fear of increasing their sense of having lost control. To alleviate this fear, you might emphasize the patient's ability to remain in control of what is discussed, as by saying: "Is there anything in your life that you do not want to talk about at this time? If there is, I won't question you about it now, unless it has direct bearing on your safety." In this way, you may make the patient less afraid of talking with you by reducing his or her fear of loss of control. Of course, you have to keep your promise. That is the reason for putting in the condition about "safety"—so that questions about such concerns as suicidal thoughts are not ruled out—and for saying "at this time" and "now," showing that the agreement is only for this interview.

Often after the patient starts talking, the excluded subject will emerge. If that happens, the doctor might say, "A few minutes ago you said that you didn't want to talk about your mother [or whoever/whatever was excluded]. Have you changed your mind?" This approach provides another chance to exert control and helps the patient to take responsibility for the decision about whether to discuss the disturbing subject.

When communication is present but incomprehensible. This kind of communication barrier is exemplified by Mr. Jermyn, who was under Dr. Transome's care (Chapter 1, pp. 4–5). When Mr. Jermyn says that demons leave his body through his belly button, Dr. Transome is tempted to set him straight. If he does so, however, Mr. Jermyn is likely to respond with anger, with withdrawal, or with something that appears to have nothing to do with demons or belly buttons or anything else. Dr. Transome has a better chance of establishing communication if he abandons the cognitive and concentrates on the affective: "That sounds as if it were upsetting to you."

Another way of coping with the apparently incomprehensible is simply to listen. What Mr. Jermyn says makes some kind of sense to himself, and Dr. Transome can try to figure it out. Dr. Transome may not "get it" at first, but his interest in the symptoms will convey caring to the patient and perhaps establish the beginning of rapport. Ultimately, with patience, the patient's previously incomprehensible comments may become understandable, and Dr. Transome may find that he can begin to communicate with his patient more intelligibly:

DR. TRANSOME [*on the fourth hospital day*]: How are you today, Mr. Jermyn?

MR. JERMYN [*for the fourth time*]: The demons keep escaping. I can't stop them. It's driving me crazy!

DR. T. [*subtly reframing the patient's comment to reflect both the patient's view ("demons") and his own (mental illness)*]: You know, it just struck me that you're trying hard to let me know how out of control everything is for you. You're afraid you're losing control and you can't stop it.

MR. J.: That's right.

DR. T.: Well, that's something we can help you with. We can help you get back in control.

MR. J.: I hope so. I can't stand this.

When communication is comprehensible but apparently irrelevant. As in the example above, "apparently" is a key word here. Much that seems irrelevant in a chronically mentally ill patient's communication may be relevant but disguised, as in the following case vignette:

> Dr. Jones visits Mr. Smith in his hospital room and asks, "How are you today?"
>
> Mr. Smith responds with a rambling commentary about the war then going on in Vietnam, including who is attacking whom, who is on the defensive, and so forth.
>
> Dr. Jones recognizes that although Mr. Smith is profoundly psychotic, he is probably responding in some way to the question, with some reference to himself. Accordingly, he asks, "Do you feel somehow under attack on the ward at this time?"
>
> Mr. Smith says that he *is* under attack, leading to a discussion about how the sources of tension might be dealt with.

The meaning of most psychotic symptoms is unfortunately much more obscure, and the physician needs to become acquainted with the patient's past and current settings, and with the influences that have molded his or her imagery and symbolism, before the idiosyncratic meaning of the patient's symptoms or behavior can begin to be understood. This search for meaning in symptoms is a challenging pursuit and, when successful, a rewarding aspect of a psychiatrist's work, as illustrated below.

Delusional communication involving the clinician. A common problem in developing rapport is that psychotic patients may include the clinician in their delusional systems, as in the following example:

> Ms. Creevy, a 28-year-old married woman with chronic schizophrenia, is agitated, pacing the floor and talking of plans to get even with her neighbors who, she says, are constantly spying on her and subject her to sadomasochistic sexual activities.
>
> Her resident, Dr. Lenville, feels that he is making progress in establishing rapport with Ms. Creevy by his empathic and interested approach. He is surprised when she tells him that she alone knows that he is Jesus Christ. When he tries to convince her that he is only a second-year resident, she smiles knowingly and asks him to call her Mary Magdalen.

The sexual nature of Ms. Creevy's delusions has forewarned Dr. Lenville that she will be likely to sexualize her relationship with him as she has done with others. In fact, there is probably no way he can avoid becoming incorporated into her delusional system, and in her current state of decompensation, "interpretations" of her behavior would be of little or no therapeutic value.

Dr. Lenville's supervisor recommends supporting Ms. Creevy's "realistic core" (i.e., the area of relatively intact ego functioning most psychotic patients retain) rather than directly confronting delusions about him. Dr. Lenville therefore focuses on realistic planning and discussion of actual occurrences with her, and frequently reminds her of the purpose of her hospitalization, as in the following interchange:

> MS. CREEVY: I know you say you're a doctor, but I know that you are Jesus Christ. You can just call me Mary Magdalen.
>
> DR. LENVILLE: Whatever we call each other, I am someone who is trying to help you. You came to the hospital because you felt afraid. I want to help you feel safer, with medication and by talking about your problems. One thing we need to think about is how to continue that help when you return home.

As Dr. Lenville learns more about Ms. Creevy, he discovers that the exacerbation of her psychosis appears to be related to her husband's frequent work-related absences from home, which she has perceived as frightening abandonments. He suspects that her delusional comments represent a wish for a relationship with a new male figure who could both "save" her and make love to her. As Ms. Creevy improves, Dr. Lenville is able to use this understanding, not to make direct interpretations, but to gently encourage the patient to discuss more realistically her feelings about her husband and her wishes for rescue.

Paranoid or overly suspicious communication. We have already pointed out how difficult it is for chronically mentally ill patients to trust the people who are trying to help them. Evidence of the distrust often emerges in paranoid delusions and hallucinations, as we have seen in the cases of Ms. Hogarth and Mr. Jermyn. In the following case, paranoid communication was initially elicited by something as innocuous as the resident's cough:

Oliver Stevenson

Oliver Stevenson, a 17-year-old adolescent with a diagnosis of paranoid schizophrenia, is admitted for evaluation and treatment. During rounds, the following exchange takes place:

> DR. FLEMING: Good morning, Oliver, how are you doing today? [*The resident coughs.*]
>
> OLIVER: You coughed.

DR. F.: I know. I seem to have caught a cold.

OLIVER: You're one of *them.*

DR. F.: One of "them"?

OLIVER: One of *them.* You're one of the people who put electrodes in my brain to control me.

DR. F.: What makes you think I am one of them?

OLIVER: Because you coughed. That's how they communicate. When they cough, I get a funny feeling. That's how I know.

DR. F.: I know that it seems like that to you. But you came to the hospital because your mind has been playing tricks on you. This is part of your illness. It upsets you because it seems so real to you. We are giving you some medication to see if that will help to keep your mind from playing tricks on you.

[*Oliver smiles slyly in a knowing way, indicating that he does not believe a word the resident is saying and that he was expecting just such an "evasive" explanation.*]

DR. F.: Are you scared of me?

OLIVER: Yeah . . .

DR. F.: There is no one here, including me, who wants to harm you. I also do not think that there are electrodes in your brain, although it seems like that to you. But, is there anything I can do to help you feel safe?

[*Oliver remains quiet.*]

DR. F.: Let me tell you what's going to happen here. I will always tell you in advance what we are planning to do and what we feel ought to be done. If you have any questions, please ask, because we want you to understand how we are trying to help you. If you get these funny feelings again, such as that I am out to hurt you, please check it out with me. I want to make sure to do what I can to make you feel safe. Eventually, I hope, you will find that you can trust me.

OLIVER [*tentatively*]: O.K.

Oliver remains unconvinced; his delusions are too powerful. Still, Dr. Fleming is beginning to establish rapport with him: she does not argue with him, and she shows respect for his experience. Her attempt to build a relationship with Oliver, along with psychotropic medication, offers the best chance to help him either to get rid of these delusions or to live with them. It would be futile for Dr. Fleming to try to avoid making Oliver suspicious, as by suppressing her coughing; a paranoid patient can always find something "suspicious" in another person's behavior and interpret it as evidence that that person is one of his or her persecutors.

Not all suspicious behavior in patients is the result of illness, as in the following example:

> Mr. Rossi has spent a long time on the ward to which Dr. Goldman has just been assigned. When she meets the patient, she introduces herself by saying, "Mr. Rossi, I am Dr. Goldman, your new doctor. Your former doctor, Dr. Clark, has been assigned to another service and he asked me to take over your treatment."
>
> Mr. Rossi looks skeptically at Dr. Goldman and says, "You may be a doctor, but you're not my doctor."
>
> Dr. Goldman wonders if Mr. Rossi is delusional.

Mr. Rossi's suspicious attitude is probably not only a symptom of psychosis, but also an expression of anger at Dr. Clark's desertion and of the patient's difficulty in accepting a stranger, the new doctor, as a confidante. Dr. Clark should have introduced Dr. Goldman personally to Mr. Rossi, but in this instance the introduction unfortunately had not taken place. Even if there had been a transfer meeting, Mr. Rossi would need time to size up his new doctor before revealing his worries and symptoms; also, even if Dr. Clark had explained the reasons for the transfer, Mr. Rossi still might have felt abandoned and therefore could have extended his resentment and distrust to the incoming Dr. Goldman. The patient will not risk another abandonment or "betrayal" until he has tested Dr. Goldman and finds that he can trust her. This testing could take months or even years, because, as we have seen, most chronically mentally ill patients have a hard time trusting anyone.

Although Mr. Rossi's distrust may disappoint Dr. Goldman, she needs to treat it as a clue to a deeper understanding of the patient, rather than as an indication for more neuroleptic medication. If Dr. Goldman feels that Mr. Rossi's resentment and distrust are out of proportion to the abruptness of the transfer, she may explore Mr. Rossi's sensitivity to changes by asking him about previous experiences with separation. In this way she may obtain important information about his past and gain insights into his modus operandi, as well as relieve her feelings of frustration.

Chronically mentally ill patients who have repeatedly related their history may be reluctant once again to recite the story of their lives and the development of their illnesses. The resident encourages good rapport by explaining why he or she is asking these questions instead of simply referring to the record. Another reason for chronic patients' distrust is stigmatization. Their unusual appearance and bizarre behavior may have elicited condescending and hostile reactions that can intensify and justify their distrust and suspiciousness.

Dr. Goldman, therefore, does not jump to the conclusion that all of Mr. Rossi's suspiciousness is paranoid. She delays assessing the meaning of this behavior until she has explored the reasons for his suspiciousness. Whatever she can do to reduce suspiciousness and to enhance trust will promote rapport in spite of the paranoia. Once patients begin to trust a clinician in one area of their life, they may be able slowly to extend that trust to allow the clinician to help with the reality testing of their delusions.

***Oliver Stevenson** (continued from p. 35)*

After several weeks in the hospital, Oliver has the following conversation with Dr. Fleming:

OLIVER: I guess you're O.K., though I still think sometimes that you're one of them.

DR. FLEMING: Oliver, in the past few weeks, I've tried to be straight with you.

OLIVER: I guess so.

DR. F.: Well, I'm being straight with you now when I tell you your mind is playing tricks on you. You can't always trust your perceptions because of your illness, and so I'd like you to trust me to help you know what's real and what's not.

Clinical Assessment of Chronically Mentally Ill Patients

The next step after establishing rapport with a patient suffering from chronic mental illness is clinical assessment.

Beyond Diagnosis: Multidimensional, Psychosocial, and Longitudinal Assessment

In the case of Mr. Jermyn in Chapter 1, Dr. Transome has stabilized the patient's acute decompensation with medication and now plans to send him home. Dr. Transome is uncomfortable about this disposition, feeling that more should be done, but he is not sure what else he can do. Dr. Transome could, however, carry out a thorough, in-depth assessment. Although DSM-III-R could be used to figure out Mr. Jermyn's diagnosis, that would not be an assessment. On the other hand, the techniques Dr. Transome has learned for making psychodynamic developmental assessments seem to apply more to neurotic patients than to Mr. Jermyn. How, then, is Dr. Transome to proceed?

In Chapter 1, we described a conceptual framework to develop an understanding of the person who suffers from chronic mental illness. This framework requires an exploration of the psychological, familial, social, environmental, and longitudinal forces that have affected the onset, course, and prognosis of the illness, and the patient's adaptation to the illness. However, for a resident attempting to assess a chronically psychotic patient who has been ill for many years and who is not a very good historian, assessment can be a daunting task.

In order to provide beginning clinicians with a sample format to guide their efforts in collecting and organizing data for the assessment of patients with chronic mental illness, a *biopsychosocial assessment protocol* has been included in Appendix A of this book. While this protocol is intended only as a guide, and other assessment formats can be used, it illustrates principles that should be applied to all assessments of chronically mentally ill individuals and their families (see Table 2–3).

The case of Mr. Jermyn illustrates this process:

Matthew Jermyn (continued from p. 5)

Mr. Jermyn had been a quiet, shy, sensitive youth and a good student but somewhat dependent and attached to his parents. Approximately 10 years ago in his senior year of high school, he became involved with a girl. After graduation, he left home to go to college, which he found

Table 2–3. General principles of individual assessment of chronically mentally ill patients

Use a multidimensional, longitudinal approach.
Assess and describe stressors.
Identify precipitating factors.
Focus on the onset of illness as a significant transforming event.
Organize data chronologically: premorbid state, onset, and course.
  Delineate course of illness.
Ascertain medication history, particularly compliance.
Focus on functioning at baseline, while patient is medication-compliant.
Ascertain if baseline is changing over time
Delineate the individual's efforts to adapt to the illness, particularly involving
  Acceptance vs. denial.
  Ability to cope with feelings.
  Realistic goals and plans.
  Level of support services needed.
Use "time line" to organize each dimension.

very stressful, and during the fall his girlfriend dropped him, apparently precipitating his first psychotic break.

He left college and was hospitalized close to home. He initially responded well to medication and to a female psychiatrist in his hometown. He saw her weekly, took his medication regularly, and lived in his parents' home for 5 years. He studied part-time at a local college and obtained a part-time job in a local market.

Five years before Mr. Jermyn's current admission, his parents moved for business reasons, which led him to terminate with his psychiatrist, because he could not contemplate living independently. Enraged at his parents and depressed by his loss, which replicated the earlier loss of his girlfriend, Mr. Jermyn responded by stopping his medicine and refusing to see the new psychiatrist to whom he had been referred. He soon decompensated, aggravating his sense of despair and worthlessness. Since then, his condition has slowly deteriorated.

As Dr. Transome uncovers Mr. Jermyn's story, he begins to see him as a real person and to realize that Mr. Jermyn's long-term noncompliance has had a purpose, which is to act out his anger while at the same time defending himself against the sadness of losing his psychiatrist. Dr. Transome decides to use the current stay in the hospital to address some of Mr. Jermyn's underlying feelings of loss and to help him to form a new attachment.

Beyond Individual Assessment: A Systematic Approach to Gathering Information

In contrast to the assessment of most other types of patients, assessment of the chronically mentally ill patient requires data from collateral sources, and not just from the patient. One usually begins with the patient, however, and then gathers data from other sources, after which one can reassess the patient to see whether the other data fit in.

The initial assessment should usually be open and unstructured to facilitate the development of rapport. Ideally, the resident encourages patients to present their problems, preoccupations, and complaints in their own way, guiding them gently to areas that need elucidation and seem pertinent. As the interview progresses, the resident can slowly begin to ask more structured questions.

Disorganized and rambling patients require more structure earlier on and may not be able to make sense of open-ended questions. With these patients, the resident may move more quickly into asking specific, concrete questions that focus on the chronology and symptoms of the illness, and the patients' view of the nature of the illness and its treatment. (For example, "Do you think you have a mental illness? If so, what is it? When did it begin? What are its symptoms? What treatment do you think you need? Do you need medication? If so, what for? If not, why do you take it?")

A physical and neurological examination is always necessary but may not have to be carried out immediately, as in the following case:

> Flavia Trenton, a 14-year-old girl, is admitted to the hospital in an agitated psychotic state, convinced that she was (and is) about to be raped and murdered. Her symptoms are so severe that she requires restraints. Because the patient's parents reported that she had no known physical illness or injury, the resident decides that little would be gained by a physical examination of a patient who could provide no assistance or information and who could easily be made worse by the process. This fact is recorded in the chart, and 36 hours later, when the patient has calmed down, a satisfactory examination is performed.

When a patient can tolerate a physical examination without feeling stressed or invaded, a psychiatrist acting in the traditional role of the physician may contribute to the patient's developing a trusting relationship.

A crucial source of information about most chronic patients is their charts, and most of these patients have extensive records of previous treatment. Although time consuming, retrieving such data is enormously important and often reveals much information that the patient will omit or forget in his or her own version. The more emergent the situation, the more it is vital for the chart to be consulted quickly.

The resident then needs to integrate the information in the chart with his or her own clinical assessment. The chart is not the only determinant of the accuracy of the assessment; symptoms—and diagnoses—change over time, and patients may reveal more to this year's resident than to last year's attending. On the other hand, it is risky to ignore or underestimate information in the chart that does not fit the current clinical picture. Chronic patients are often adept at concealing or minimizing their psychotic symptoms and at discounting the severity of their illnesses and need for medication. For example, the apparently nonpsychotic patient with a 10-year history of schizophrenia documented in the chart may still need his fluphenazine, even though he seems to be functioning well now. Although it may be possible for a resident to discover the "true" diagnosis that everyone has missed, it is at least as likely that what everyone else has picked up is still part of the picture.

After reviewing the chart, it is usually best not to confront patients bluntly with information they have not revealed, at least until solid rapport is established. Patients may feel uncomfortable or angry if they are "hit over the head" with material about which they are ashamed, guilty, or in denial. The resident can instead use what he or she has learned from the chart as a guide to assess patients' ability to perceive their illness accurately.

The next step in gathering data involves talking to the family. Taking a careful history of the patient from the family can help them feel involved and validated, thus facilitating the development of rapport.

Finally, the resident needs to make sure that all involved clinicians are contacted, including case managers, residential counselors, therapists, and medicating psychiatrists. Each may have unique data to contribute about the course of the patient's illness and response to treatment. At the same time that this information is gathered for assessment purposes, these clinicians can begin to be involved in treatment planning and, for hospitalized patients, in preparations for discharge.

In summary, therefore, the process of individual assessment of the chronically mentally ill patient involves not just talking to the individual patient, but systematically contacting and gathering data from the chart, and contacting and obtaining information from the family and from other clinicians. The speed with which data must be gathered depends on the acuteness of the case; even in less acute cases, these data are needed to fill in information that the patient cannot provide. Once a complete picture is obtained, the resident may be able to respond to the patient more as a "whole person" and use his or her empathic understanding to facilitate treatment planning.

3

Engagement and Assessment of the Family

In the vignette in Chapter 1, Dr. Transome was overwhelmed by the demands and needs of Matthew Jermyn's parents. As a result, he cut short his initial meeting with them and avoided them during the remainder of Matthew's hospitalization. If, however, Dr. Transome had engaged and assessed Mr. Jermyn as described in Chapter 2, he might have been more sensitive to the needs and experiences of the Jermyn family. He might even have discovered, to his surprise, that he looked forward to meetings with Matthew's parents.

In any case, Dr. Transome would probably have discovered that the parents were no less distraught and burnt out at the second meeting than they were at the first. The scenario may well have played as follows:

Matthew Jermyn (continued from p. 39)

The parents continue to plead for an extended respite from the care of their son and argue vociferously for a long hospitalization. Dr. Transome begins to feel pressured, defensive, and irritated, and he is tempted once again to ask the parents to leave. But when he puts himself in their shoes and thinks about how he would feel if a similar tragedy had befallen a member of his own family, he finds it easier to recognize their pain and guilt, and their conflict about continuing to take care of Matthew.

Dr. Transome says to the Jermyns: "It must be awful for you both to see Matthew the way he is, and to feel so hopeless about his condition. I know you love him, but it must be so difficult to keep trying to take care of him." This empathic comment softens the Jermyns, and Mrs. Jermyn begins to cry. Dr. Transome continues: "I'm just beginning to get to know Matthew, and I know how difficult his illness has been, particularly since he lost his former psychiatrist. I am trying to see if there may be a way we can help Matthew to get back on track."

This response allows the Jermyns to communicate more openly with Dr. Transome about the history of their son's illness and about their own feelings and concerns. Dr. Transome sidesteps the conflict about Matthew's length of stay, stating only that it is too soon to predict the length of the hospitalization and that he needs first to learn more about the issues the family is facing.

Dr. Transome's difficulty with Matthew's parents is similar to that faced by Dr. Holt with Ms. Hogarth's mother, and by Dr. Lyon with Ms. DeBarry's mother. But because family members are crucial caregivers for many chronically mentally ill patients, their involvement in the process of assessment and treatment is essential. As with the Jermyns, the intensity of their distress may be so great that they create barriers to receiving the help that they seek. Our purpose in this chapter is to help residents to develop specific techniques for overcoming those barriers, for engaging families successfully, and for accurately assessing their problems and needs.

Engagement of Families

Dr. Transome's experience with Matthew Jermyn's family illustrates that the same basic principles of building rapport, using empathic communication, and ensuring safety apply to the engagement of families as apply to the engagement of individuals.

Building Rapport

A barrier to establishing rapport with the families of chronically mentally ill patients is the tendency of residents to expect more of families than of patients, and thus to feel impatient when families have difficulty collaborating with treatment. Some families are too anxious to be objective, while others may persist in denying the illness.

Families' needs may feel overwhelmingly burdensome to already burdened residents, especially when family members make demands or ask questions to which residents do not know how to respond. Some families, who may be angry because of disappointments with previous treatment efforts, may be seen as unfairly attacking the residents' competence.

In some cases, residents may feel drawn in to taking the patient's "side" against the family, blaming them for contributing to the patient's illness or interfering with the recovery process. Family members may be divided about what is "best" for the patient, and residents may find themselves caught in the middle of the family conflict.

Finally, residents may feel unable to bear the pain and despair that families must face, particularly if they find little support from their colleagues.

To overcome these difficulties, it is usually helpful to follow guidelines similar to those outlined for working with individuals (see Table 3–1). Thus, the resident can start by imagining himself or herself in the family's predicament, asking: "How would I behave if my child were mentally ill? How would my parents behave if I were mentally ill? What limits would *I* be able to set with my own relative?"

The guilt, shame, helplessness, hopelessness, and frustration that family members often feel interfere with their ability to participate in treatment. Treating the family as "normal" people puts them at ease by creating a friendly, casual, and somewhat informal atmosphere. Treating them with respect, courtesy, and dignity, especially when their behavior is undignified, helps them to become collaborators who need to learn new skills for managing their relative's illness. Adversarial conflict is to be avoided, even if it means giving in to some of a family's requests in the interest of maintaining rapport. If such acquiescence is simply not possible, the resident should communicate sincere regret and seek other ways of responding to the family's needs.

Often the perception that you are willing to extend yourself to help is more important than the reality of what you can do. One should try to refer to the family's behavior in positive terms, even when it is maladaptive, as a reflection of their concern for the patient and their difficulty accepting the pain of his or her illness. A family that "sabotages" a treatment plan, for example, may be telling us that they are not ready to accept the painful implications of following the plan. If possible,

Table 3–1. Guidelines for establishing rapport with families of chronically mentally ill patients

Imagine yourself in the family's predicament.
Treat the family respectfully as "normal people" in a traumatic situation.
Avoid adversarial conflict.
Frame the family's behavior as a reflection of their concern for the patient.
Avoid implication of blame; avoid labeling or "pathologizing" family behavior.
Listen to affective tone as well as content.
Communicate empathic understanding clearly.
Focus on developing collaboration in managing the patient's illness.

any implication of blame or criticism of the family is to be avoided. Families already feel guilty and ashamed, and adding to these feelings is likely to lead to more defensiveness. The family can be told explicitly that the basic cause of mental illness is biological, not bad parenting, and that they should learn how not to blame themselves for what has happened. To get this message across, residents need to avoid judgmental labeling or "pathologizing" of families, as by using such terms as "schizophrenogenic" or "double-binding," both openly and in their own thoughts.

The resident needs to listen to affective tone as well as to content, and to communicate empathic understanding in clear, simple language. Families appreciate openness and willingness to listen, and they will accept these qualities in you even though they know you are inexperienced. As an example, you might say to the parents of a young man who has just had his first episode of schizophrenia: "I know you are terribly concerned about your son's future, and I share that concern with you. We do know he has a very serious illness, but we don't know yet how it will come out. All I can say is that we'll work with you as closely as possible and keep you informed every step of the way."

The following brief vignette illustrates the initial engagement of a family whose son has had a second psychotic break:

> The parents of John Marlowe, a 17-year-old schizophrenic young man hospitalized for the second time, ask to see Dr. Spencer. John had first been hospitalized a year previously and had been reluctant to enter into treatment; before the present admission, he had discontinued his medication. Both parents, the patient, and two younger siblings come to the appointment.
>
> The mother, speaking in a trembling voice, leads off: "We are all terribly worried about John. All of us, including John, are beginning to think that he may be more seriously ill than we thought. It seems he can't think straight without the medication. We all feel we need to know his diagnosis."
>
> Dr. Spencer tells them that he shares their concerns and that, to the best of his knowledge, their son is suffering from schizophrenia. They are very upset at this news, and Dr. Spencer spends the rest of the meeting empathizing with their feelings and answering their questions about John's diagnosis, treatment, and prognosis. John is especially upset at first, and during the next several days he needs a good deal of reassurance.

Although an evasive answer to the question about diagnosis would have spared the patient some distress and might have saved some time for the resident, it probably would have either confirmed the family's and the patient's fears that schizophrenia was a disorder so dreadful that it could not be discussed, or strengthened the family's denial of the seriousness of the condition. Either way would have made it more difficult for patient and family to face realistically the tasks of understanding and care.

Most parents whose hopes and expectations have been cruelly dashed by their child's chronic mental illness have done everything they could for their child. Now they need more than just information; they need an ongoing supportive relationship with a clinician who can assist them with planning for the future and with the reestablishment of realistic expectations, while at the same time being supportive during recurrent crises caused by their child's relapses. In this chapter we will discuss ways to recognize when a patient's grieving family needs such support. (The details of this relationship will be described in Chapter 8.)

Overcoming Barriers to Engaging the Family

The process of engagement of families seldom proceeds smoothly because of barriers generated by the patient, such as refusal to give permission to contact the family, and those generated by the family. Family members often are so overwhelmed by the pain of the patient's illness that they behave in ways that make it hard for them to accept or receive help. Some families refuse to accept the patient's diagnosis and so resist engagement. Others may be very needy, making many demands and insisting on involvement in every detail of treatment. Still other families may be overwhelmed or exhausted, unable to expend the energy to be involved constructively. Finally, there are families whose internal conflicts and disagreements interfere with family members' ability to collaborate with treatment. Once the patient has agreed to the family's involvement, specific techniques are required to overcome each of these barriers.

The Patient's Barrier: Refusal to Give Permission to Contact the Family

Mr. Milton, a 36-year-old, physically disabled, unemployed, and recently divorced outpatient, has been referred by the physician who made the physical disability determination after Mr. Milton had been injured at work 2 years before. Mr. Milton is anxious and afraid that "the system is going to get me." After the psychiatrist establishes rapport, the patient confides that he has many enemies because of the military secrets he knows from his Navy days. He refuses to talk about his illness, his hospitalizations, and certain periods of his life. He does not wish to live with nearby relatives because of the "way they treated me earlier in my life."

To find out more about Mr. Milton's past, the psychiatrist suggests a meeting with Mr. Milton's relatives in which the patient could participate if he wishes. The patient, however, adamantly refuses to give permission to contact his relatives. The psychiatrist accepts his decision and declares that he will work with him as well as he can.

Although Mr. Milton is somewhat suspicious of the psychiatrist, he keeps returning for treatment and begins slowly to trust him. He gradually reveals a delusional system that includes fears of communism and nuclear war. After 6 months he confesses to the psychiatrist that as a child he had been sexually abused and severely beaten. It then becomes clear why Mr. Milton is unwilling to allow the psychiatrist to contact his family.

In this case the psychiatrist honors the patient's refusal to give permission to communicate with his relatives. The psychiatrist's restraint pays off and contributes to the building of a trusting therapeutic relationship.

It is not always possible, however, to accede to the patient's wishes:

Nancy Heathcliff is a 27-year-old woman with a 6-year history of recurrent psychotic illness. Following two psychotic episodes in rapid succession, she has done well in outpatient treatment as long as she has maintained her neuroleptic medication. She lives alone, works as a sales clerk, takes evening college courses, and leads an acceptable, though limited, social life. Her family, however, maintains periodic contacts with her.

Because she has been stable for nearly 5 years, and because she is concerned about tardive dyskinesia, Ms. Heathcliff requests a reduction in her antipsychotic medication, to which her therapist agrees. When the dose is about half its former level, Ms. Heathcliff begins to experience prodromal symptoms of a recurrent psychosis. The therapist reminds her of the concerns both had expressed when the dose reduction was first considered. The patient is nevertheless convinced that her symptoms are insignificant, and when the therapist suggests that her parents should be involved in the decision, Ms. Heathcliff insists that confidentiality be maintained.

Over the succeeding weeks, while Ms. Heathcliff's condition is becoming gradually worse, she adamantly resists the psychiatrist's suggestions for the medication to be increased or for her parents to be involved. Finally, Ms. Heathcliff phones the therapist to inform him, in a confused and disorganized torrent of words, that she has resigned from her job, is discontinuing her medication, and is terminating her treatment. She repeats her insistence that her parents should not be informed of her actions.

Nevertheless, after indicating his intentions to Ms. Heathcliff, the therapist phones her parents and explains the situation, because he is concerned that Ms. Heathcliff might be in imminent danger. He suggests that they visit their daughter and, if she seems to be in serious trouble, that they bring her to the hospital emergency room where they could all review the situation. At this meeting Ms. Heathcliff agrees to hospitalization. Once she is in the hospital and responding to medication, the psychiatrist explains why he had to contact her parents, and she thanks him for his concern.

On an inpatient unit, patients who refuse to allow contact with their families may respond to a combination of empathy and firm limits:

Matthew Jermyn (continued from p. 44)

When Dr. Transome's patient, Mr. Jermyn, was first admitted, he refused to allow contact with his family. He was informed that family involvement was an essential part of his treatment, but that he had time to make up his mind. He was also informed that he could not go home on passes unless a family meeting was held. As Mr. Jermyn becomes less psychotic and more trusting of staff, he decides to allow contact with his family in order to go out.

As these case vignettes illustrate, there are no simple answers to the question of what to do when a psychotic patient refuses to permit the therapist to contact the family. Whenever possible, a patient's wishes should be respected in order to maintain good rapport; however, when a patient lacks the judgment to take the steps necessary to secure his or her safety, the psychiatrist has no choice and must initiate measures even against the patient's expressed wishes. Such a decision should be discussed with the patient, who should be allowed to retain as much control over the family contact as possible, as by deciding who will be present for the initial meeting and, to the extent possible, what will or will not be discussed.

Family Barriers

The family in denial. Fortunately, most patients do not object to their doctors' talking to their families. But sometimes the family is reluctant to talk because to do so would threaten their denial of the seriousness of the illness. Denial is most frequent in families during the relative's first psychotic episode, as in the following case vignette. In some instances, however, denial seems to harden with each psychotic break.

> Robert Bligh, a 21-year-old college student, is being hospitalized for the first time with a psychotic episode. His middle-class parents had been aware of his increasingly disorganized and bizarre behavior for several weeks, but failed to take any action until he began to speak incoherently, broke some furniture, and was taken to the hospital.
>
> The parents appear overwhelmed by guilt and appalled by the severity of their son's illness. They say they had suspected that there was something wrong with him but had hoped his symptoms were "just a form of adolescent rebellion."
>
> The attempts to educate Mr. Bligh's parents about his illness and treatment are thwarted by their continuing grief and denial. His mother insists that his problems are caused by junk food, and she brings a number of pamphlets to the hospital to support her convictions. Eventually she is permitted to participate in planning her son's diet on condition that she agree to allow him to use medication. As she participates in the treatment process, she gradually permits herself to be educated about her son's illness. To make this possible, the clinician has had to listen patiently as the mother discussed her son's diet at length, but this is the beginning of a long-lasting collaboration that will greatly facilitate the patient's rehabilitation.

This vignette illustrates the importance of meeting the family members where they are. Permitting—and even supporting—the mother's involvement in Mr. Bligh's illness on her own terms will facilitate the development of long-lasting rapport.

The angry, resistant family. Engagement of the family can take much longer to achieve, as in the following example:

> Jill Tremayne is 25 years old when she is hospitalized for her fifth schizoaffective episode in a little over 6 years. Ms. Tremayne has been a source of great pride and hope to her parents. She graduated at the top of her high school class and obtained a college scholarship, and her athletic good looks have made her a popular figure in their small town. Unwilling to accept the seriousness of her illness, the family has told Ms. Tremayne to discontinue medication and psychotherapy as soon as her symptoms abate, and they have angrily resisted all attempts by staff to educate them about her illness, as in this exchange from a family meeting:
>
> > MOTHER: You people are wrong about Jill. I now know what has caused her confusion. It's all the smoking she's been doing.
> >
> > M.D.: Smoking marijuana?
> >
> > MOTHER: Oh no, it's cigarettes. It's clear to all of us that cigarettes have caused the trouble.

Despite repeated rebuffs, the staff has kept trying to help the family accept the fact of Ms. Tremayne's chronic illness. Staff members let the family know that their pain is understood and that their resistance, while not helpful, is understandable. For example, one resident, when confronted angrily by the Tremaynes, tells them the following:

> I know that we disagree about Jill's diagnosis and need for ongoing medication, but I don't feel that we need to argue. I understand your pain; if Jill were in my family, I might be saying exactly what you are. I wish you were right and Jill wouldn't need medication after discharge. But whatever happens, we'll try to help all of your family get through the crisis.

After the fifth hospitalization the denial begins to crack, and the Tremaynes begin, hesitantly and painfully, to come to terms with the severity of their daughter's illness. This recognition is followed by a period of demoralization and depression, but with a good deal of support the family regains some hope. Since then, Ms. Tremayne has been able to avoid hospitalization, although she has had some shaky periods.

Even though it took years before this family was able to accept Ms. Tremayne's illness, the residents who met with them at each hospitalization contributed toward her eventual reasonably good outcome, as their cumulative effort finally paid off. Residents in similar situations may not always see the results of their efforts, but eventually their input, together with the efforts of their predecessors and successors, will usually bear fruit.

Families such as the Tremaynes are difficult to manage even for experienced therapists. Their blatant and apparently irrational denial may appear to be a kind of sabotage set up to make the resident fail, and the family's desperate efforts to maintain their equilibrium in the face of their family member's devastating illness may not be appreciated. As in the case of Mr. Jermyn in Chapter 1, the resident may then begin to avoid the family and perhaps the patient as well, which could lead to the patient's premature discharge. At this juncture, the resident, often with the help of a compassionate supervisor, needs to work on accepting and understanding his or her anger without acting on it.

The needy, highly involved family. Another type of family that may arouse angry feelings is the needy, involved family, as illustrated by the following case:

After a long period of behavior problems at school, 16-year-old James Conrad suffers an acute psychotic illness. He responds quickly to medication and is placed in a treatment school, where he is maintained on a daily dose of haloperidol. He does well until he goes home for the Christmas holiday, at which time he becomes acutely psychotic, requiring rehospitalization. It soon becomes clear that Jim had gotten his medications only sporadically at home, although the school nurse had sent a note to his parents instructing them about the dosage schedule.

The staff has been frustrated by the Conrads' apparent inability to grasp the nature of Jim's illness, and by Jim's mother's almost hourly calls to ask about her son. She has often slipped into Jim's room after visiting hours to rub his back or to rock him in her lap, irritating the staff, who begin to talk of her as being "responsible for Jim's illness."

Meanwhile, the resident in charge of Jim's case tries to engage the parents and understand them. She discovers that Mr. and Mrs. Conrad emigrated from southern Europe 10 years earlier. Mr. Conrad has integrated into American society much better than Mrs. Conrad. He speaks excellent English and holds a responsible professional position, while she speaks broken English and spends most of her time alone at home, with Jim having been her only company until he left for school. As the resident recognizes that Mrs. Conrad's loneliness is interfering with her ability to relinquish Jim's care to the treatment team, she begins to feel empathy for Mrs. Conrad's pain rather than anger at her "overinvolvement."

A staff meeting is held with the parents to develop a strategy to help Mrs. Conrad to deal with her distress and to learn to help her son. A nurse is asked to work with Mrs. Conrad through regular telephone calls and frequent meetings. With support, Mrs. Conrad's loneliness and homesickness are addressed, and she is helped to arrange contact with immigrant groups in her area. Only now can she respond to the staff's educational efforts.

Whole families—or, as in this case, a particular family member—may be highly enmeshed with a patient for reasons that have little to do with the illness. These reasons include the desire to feel like a needed parent, the avoidance of loneliness or emptiness, and the wish to overcome guilt for not having prevented the illness. The family members' efforts to keep involved with the patient during treatment are often resented by the treatment team. This resentment may result in efforts to pry the patient loose from the family, which only leads the family to intensify their efforts to stay involved. It is more constructive to take the time to get to know the family, empathize with their concerns, and provide them with a supportive context in which to remain involved.

The burned-out family. A long-standing chronic illness can be exceedingly wearing on the family. An earlier GAP Report (No. 119, *A Family Affair: Helping Families Cope with Mental Illness*) details the enormous burden and sadness families experience when a mentally ill relative lives at home. Under this type of stress, families like the Jermyns often become "burned out" and seek to initiate or extend hospitalization in order to obtain relief. Such families often have little energy to expend on being involved in treatment, and they may seem to the resident to be trying to "dump" the patient, as in the following example:

Dale Wharton

Mr. and Mrs. Wharton come to the psychiatric emergency room with their 22-year-old son, Dale, who has a 2-year history of schizophrenia. They complain that Dale is "worse"; they are afraid of him and want him back in the hospital. Although Dale's symptoms have improved on medication, he has never been in complete remission. His roaming by night, and his bizarre behavior, threats of violence, temper tantrums, and seclusiveness by day, are sources of continuing stress to his parents. They have never quite accepted their son's illness and so have difficulty engaging with the treatment staff or learning how to set limits on their son.

The resident interviews Dale Wharton and his parents and reviews the clinic chart. He concludes that Dale's symptoms are no worse than they have been for some time and that hospitalization is not indicated. He suggests that the parents attempt to work with their son's therapist to understand his illness better and find ways to minimize the stress on themselves. They react angrily to this recommendation and reemphasize that their son should be admitted. The resident sticks to his views, pointing out that Dale himself does not wish to be admitted, and then repeats his recommendations. The parents leave angrily with their son.

That evening, they reappear with a police officer and a commitment order. They say that upon returning home their son became agitated and attempted to strike his father. The resident now has no choice but to admit him.

Later the resident realizes that he has been struggling with the family rather than engaging them. In retrospect, he thinks that he might have taken a more empathic stance by recognizing the legitimacy of their perception of the lack of control and safety in their home.

A dilemma for the resident in this type of situation is that the family and the patient are in conflict, so maintaining rapport with both patient and family simultaneously may be difficult. Usually, however, the patient and family's overt anger is balanced by an underlying wish to find a way to resolve their conflict. If the resident can find a way to ally with this wish on both sides, he can usually maintain rapport with all parties. For example, in the Whartons' case, the resident might address Dale as follows:

M.D.: Mr. Wharton, your parents want you to be hospitalized. They feel things aren't working at home. What do you think?

MR. WHARTON: They're wrong. Everything's fine. They want me to be a puppet, but I won't let them.

M.D.: It sounds pretty tense for you at home as well. Do you want to keep on living with them?

MR. W.: I want my own place, but they won't give me the money.

M.D.: So you're stuck with them for now.

MR. W.: Yeah.

M.D.: Maybe if you go into the hospital now, we can work out some of the tensions at home for you as well. Besides, I think they really mean to have you committed this time.

MR. W.: They wouldn't do that.

PARENTS: Oh yes we would!

MR. W. [*seeing a united front*]: Well, O.K., then, I'll go—for a while.

The family with internal conflict. In previous examples, we have spoken about engaging "the family" as if it were a single entity. Actually, family members may disagree with each other as well as with the patient or the doctor. Engaging such families requires tact and even-handedness, as illustrated in the following case:

James William is a 22-year-old single man who has been admitted to the hospital with a 1-year history of social withdrawal, suspiciousness, increasing hostility to his parents and siblings, and, finally, paranoid delusions. The patient's difficulty in his relationship with his mother is evident in family meetings, where he has lost his temper with her over trivial or imaginary matters. His mother, in turn, has reported increasing alarm as the tension between them has grown over the past months.

In spite of some improvement with medication, Mr. William continues to be enraged at his mother, and the treatment team has become increasingly concerned about the wisdom and safety of Mr. William's returning to his family home. The team therefore recommends that he be discharged to a nearby halfway house, a plan his mother endorses with relief. Both the patient and his father oppose the plan, however, adamantly insisting that Mr. William should return home, and, after considerable discussion, the team reluctantly allows the patient to do so.

Two months later, the patient is rehospitalized after a suicidal gesture. On readmission, his parents report that the tension between Mr. William and his mother had gradually increased since his return home until it reached explosive proportions. All of the family members now agree to Mr. William's placement in the halfway house.

Mr. William's alliance with his son rather than with his wife suggests that the son's anger may reflect an underlying marital conflict. However, exploring this possibility at this juncture could scare the family off rather than build an alliance. So instead of taking sides, the team supported the family in its ambivalence as a unit and respected its process for resolving the internal dispute. Thus, even though the members of the family could not agree to follow the team's recommendation, they remained involved. This made it easier for Mrs. William to give her husband some space to make up his mind, and for Mr. William and his father to change their decision when the situation at home deteriorated.

Ensuring Safety for the Family

In Chapter 2, we spoke about the importance of preventing violence and self-injury in order to create a safe context for a treatment relationship to develop. Ensuring safety is equally important when engaging the family. If the family feels unsafe with the patient—even though no one else does—treatment cannot proceed until the family's concerns are evaluated and appropriate measures are taken to ensure family members' safety.

The case of the Whartons, described earlier, illustrates this point. The Whartons felt that their son's behavior was out of control in their home and were concerned about his potential for violence. But because in his initial evaluation the resident found Mr. Wharton to be calm and only minimally disorganized, he discounted the family's concern.

Thus, some chronic patients who are dangerous at home seem to be in control in the presence of a clinician or in a treatment setting. Even when the resident feels that the family is contributing to the tension, the home situation may still be unsafe and the danger must be addressed.

The situation with the Whartons had progressed to the extent that only hospitalization could help the family feel in control and protected. In most instances, however, a resident can ensure safety by empowering the family to enforce reasonable limits, with backup guaranteed by the resident.

For example, once Dale is in the hospital, the resident might say to the Whartons the following:

> When Dale returns home, we want to help you make sure that your home will be safe for all of you. That means that we need to let Dale know that certain kinds of behavior, like violence, threats, or temper outbursts, will not be tolerated, just as they are not tolerated here in the hospital.
>
> If Dale's behavior scares you, you should call the emergency service immediately, and we will arrange for Dale to be evaluated in

the emergency room. This will let him know that you intend to keep things under control. Although he may complain, like most patients he is likely to feel reassured when he sees that others care enough to prevent him from behaving destructively.

If the emergency room gives you a hard time, have them call me, and I will back you up. We will also work out a written treatment plan for Dale that can be kept on file in the emergency room for reference. Once we can help you to guarantee some safety in your home, we can begin to work on the longer-term treatment issues.

Clinical Assessment of the Families of Chronically Mentally Ill Patients

The next step after engagement with the families of chronically mentally ill patients is assessment.

Longitudinal Psychosocial Assessment

At the beginning of this chapter, we left Dr. Transome in the process of beginning an assessment of Mr. Jermyn's parents. Dr. Transome is pleased to have found a way to engage the Jermyns, but he is uncertain about how to proceed with their clinical evaluation. His knowledge of family systems theory is sketchy, although he recognizes Matthew as being the so-called "identified patient" in the family system. Dr. Transome is concerned that the family might feel criticized or blamed if he asks too many pointed questions, but he is not sure how else he can find out what he needs to know about them to be most useful in planning treatment.

He can start by exploring the impact of the illness on the family, paying particular attention to their efforts to accept, bear, and adapt to the illness (see Table 3–2).

The history of the family's adaptation to the illness leads to an understanding of current issues: the family's concerns about the patient's treatment, compliance, and progress, and their own roles and needs. Do they feel safe and in control, or scared and overwhelmed? Are they able to enforce medication compliance or participation in treatment? If the patient lives with the family, do family members provide money, rides, cigarettes, and so forth, and do they require any level of performance by the patient in return? Does the family have their own supports, such as extended family, therapists, and/or support groups? Collecting and organizing this information will allow the resident to put the family's long-term struggle with the illness into perspective, and permit the development of a specific treatment plan.

Table 3–2. Issues in family assessment

Address immediate crisis concerns.
Assess preillness family context.
Identify impact of illness on adaptation.
Explore current family stresses.
Maintain longitudinal and chronological focus.

The Process of Family Assessment

It is advisable for the resident to begin, and in many cases to complete, the assessment process by meeting with the family without the patient. Although it is desirable to involve all of the relatives in the initial assessment, some relatives may be too burned out, frightened, or angry to participate.

The family needs to be at ease during the assessment. Because families expect to be criticized for their imagined or real shortcomings or failures, the resident will facilitate more open sharing of information by explicitly telling the family that they have done the best they could.

While the assessment *protocol* begins with the onset of illness, the assessment *process* will usually begin with an empathic exploration of the family's current concerns. Once the family feel that their immediate needs are understood, they will be more willing to move on to provide background, particularly if the resident's attitude is consistently warm, neutral, and accepting. The assessment allows the family to reveal any irrational fears, ideas, and concerns; because confronting their irrationality too early only causes them to go underground, it is best to resist the impulse to argue with family members who say things that are outlandish, misinformed, or provocative.

A return to Dr. Transome and the Jermyn family shows how that family assessment turned out.

Matthew Jermyn (continued from p. 49)

After listening empathically to the Jermyns' painful account of their frustration with their son and his repeated noncompliance, Dr. Transome begins to explore their view of the onset and course of their son's illness. It soon becomes apparent that they feel overwhelmed by guilt and are plagued by the belief that they caused the illness:

DR. TRANSOME: So, how did Matthew's illness begin?

MR. JERMYN: We didn't know what to do. He was such a sensitive kid, you know, that we felt he needed protection. Then, when he went away to college—I guess he couldn't handle it.

MRS. JERMYN [*tearful*]: He was always a good kid. We took care of him, maybe too much care. We should have pushed him more . . .

DR. T.: It sounds like you both feel you're to blame?

MR. J.: Well, I mean, we know it's an illness. We've been told that, and all. But we can't help wondering. If we'd only . . . you know.

DR. T.: I don't feel you're to blame. However, it does sound as if you both need some help to feel less guilty. Now, what can you tell me about Matthew's high school girl friend?

As Dr. Transome moves through Matthew's history, he finds that the Jermyns' guilt intensified after the family move that preceded their son's decompensation. Currently, they are furious at Matthew for his obnoxious behavior at home and his failure to comply with treatment, but they also feel sorry for him and responsible for his plight. Because of their conflicting feelings, they cannot find a way to set any limits. They can only hope the hospital will keep him "for a while," but they cannot bear to think about refusing to allow him to come home.

Once Dr. Transome hears their story, he sees them as caring, responsible parents, and his anger at them for wanting to "dump" Matthew melts. Dr. Transome is not sure how to help them, but he feels that if he could help them to feel less guilty, they might be able to set more limits and enforce their son's treatment compliance. Dr. Transome begins to feel more hopeful about the outcome.

This vignette illustrates how a family assessment can illuminate the reasons for a family's maladaptive behavior, as well as provide data for the clinician to begin to develop a treatment plan. Treatment planning for chronically mentally ill patients also involves community resources, programs, and systems. In the next chapter we will discuss the engagement and assessment of various treatment systems.

4

Engagement and Assessment of the Treatment System

Mary Hogarth (continued from p. 30)

Ms. Hogarth, as described at the beginning of Chapter 2, has just been admitted to the care of Dr. Lincoln, a resident on the inpatient unit. Although Dr. Lincoln appreciates the work Dr. Holt has done in engaging Ms. Hogarth and her mother, he has many reservations about working with Mary.

First of all, he is concerned about how she will fit into the ward milieu, anticipating that her bizarre behavior might not be welcomed in the inpatient groups. He is also worried that he might be pressured by the nursing staff about Ms. Hogarth's compliance with unit rules. For a moment, Dr. Lincoln wishes he were back in his medical internship, where the ward system had been simple and straightforward. Here on the psychiatry unit, by contrast, the system of milieu care is complex and the lines of authority are unclear.

Dr. Lincoln is also unsure about how to go about discharging Ms. Hogarth. As a chronic patient who has been around the mental health system for years, Ms. Hogarth has been in and out of contact with many programs and caregivers. Dr. Lincoln is unfamiliar with the community system and with how to assess Ms. Hogarth's involvement with community resources in order to plan her discharge; in Dr. Lincoln's internship the social worker took care of discharge planning.

Dr. Lincoln considers some of the areas in which planning might be needed: Ms. Hogarth's vocational day program, her aftercare, her residence, her income and health insurance, and her support systems. If Ms. Hogarth requires commitment, Dr. Lincoln will also have to deal with the legal system.

Dr. Lincoln's concerns are familiar to residents beginning to work with chronically mentally ill patients. Patients with chronic mental illness can rarely be helped by doctor-patient contact alone. Other clinicians, programs, and agencies—that is, other systems of care—are a necessary part of the treatment. To work with chronic patients successfully, residents need to learn to engage and assess the particular systems with which each patient is involved. Furthermore, residents also need to learn to engage and assess the systems with which they are involved—their own clinic or ward, their own catchment area service network, and so on. The more adept residents become in system skills in their own system, the more success they will have in adapting the system to the needs of particular patients.

In this chapter, we will consider specific techniques for engaging and assessing the three major systems with which residents come in contact: the *ward (or clinic) system*, the *catchment area service system* (i.e., the community system), and the *legal system.*

The Ward System

Conflict

The unit on which Dr. Lincoln works has a strong milieu program in which participation in a daily schedule of groups and activities is required for all patients. A problem arises when Ms. Hogarth, who has now been somewhat restabilized on antipsychotic medication, refuses to attend her assigned therapeutic group meeting. When the nurses encourage her to attend, she lashes out angrily. The nurses are upset and approach the head nurse, who in turn approaches Dr. Lincoln:

NURSE: Ms. Hogarth refuses to go to group.

DR. LINCOLN [*defensively*]: So what can I do about it?

NURSE: Make her go.

DR. L.: Even if I could, why should I?

NURSE: It's the unit policy.

DR. L.: But doesn't she have a right to refuse?

NURSE: We can't allow her to get away with that.

DR. L. [*arbitrarily*]: Look, she's my patient, and I feel she's too sick to go. O.K.?

The nurse walks away, leaving Dr. Lincoln feeling upset but satisfied at having defended his patient from the system. The head nurse, however, is furious at Dr. Lincoln's insensitivity to the needs of the team and the unit and decides to complain about him to the Chief. She also will be less likely to cover for Dr. Lincoln if he has any problems in the future. The nurse says to herself that she will try harder in the future to keep chronic patients like Ms. Hogarth from being admitted.

In this example of an unsuccessful approach to a ward system problem, Dr. Lincoln quickly sets up an adversarial relationship and uses his medical authority to "win." In winning the battle, however, he loses the war and sets up a more difficult climate for himself and the patient.

Collaboration

The key to a successful approach, as in the following illustration, is to avoid the adversarial stance:

> NURSE [*angrily*]: Ms. Hogarth refuses to go to group.
>
> DR. LINCOLN [*empathically*]: That's annoying. What's going on?
>
> [*The nurse fills in the details.*]
>
> DR. L.: I agree with you that we can't let her violate unit rules, but I'm not sure I know what to do. How have we handled these situations in the past?
>
> [*The nurse, feeling less tense, provides Dr. Lincoln with the necessary information.*]
>
> DR. L.: Well, that's helpful. I'll talk to Ms. Hogarth now to see if I can figure out what's going on and see if she needs more meds. Then let's see if we can come up with some kind of compromise. Maybe she could come to each group for 15 minutes, and then she can be restricted to her room if she wants to leave.

In this successful approach, Dr. Lincoln focuses on his alliance with the nurse and the unit. He uses the pronouns "we" and "us" rather than "you" versus "me." Instead of jumping to conclusions, he takes the time to gather information about the patient's behavior and about unit traditions. He then validates the concerns of both patient and staff, reinforces the need for limits, and recommends a joint decision. In this process, Dr. Lincoln actually encourages a supportive alliance that will make the team more helpful to Ms. Hogarth in the long run, and one that may challenge her to be more responsible for her behavior. Moreover, the development of a successful alliance will encourage the team to feel better about working with chronic patients in the future.

There is always a "bottom line" at which the patient has the responsibility for complying with the system's needs and rules or else must be subject to sanctions, which can include discharge or transfer. Compliance thus becomes a therapeutic issue for the patient. Paradoxically, the more validation that is given to the team's or unit's limits, the less stringently these limits are likely to be needed and applied.

To implement this approach, Dr. Lincoln needs to know the parameters of treatment on the unit. Appendix B provides a list of questions whose answers clarify treatment policies; these questions are applicable to hospitals, clinics, or other structured treatment settings. It is also important for the resident to know who has the authority and responsibility for carrying out these policies—in other words, the clinical and administrative organizational structure of the treatment setting.

A Graceful Retreat

Mary Hogarth (continued from p. 59)

Ms. Hogarth has kept on violating the unit rules and the terms of her contract. Dr. Lincoln is tempted to be lenient, but other members of the team want her discharged immediately. Realizing that proposing his unpopular plan would lead to disagreement within the team and would place him in the position of being unsupportive of unit rules, Dr. Lincoln decides to check out his plan with the head nurse and the unit medical director. Both are sympathetic to Ms. Hogarth's plight but firm in their conviction that she needs to be discharged, especially since her behavior is undermining the treatment of other patients on the unit.

Learning to work with teams is part of the challenge and excitement of psychiatry; gaining the support and allegiance of the various teams the resident will work with will make his or her work with persons with chronic mental illness easier and more gratifying. Many of the same concerns apply to the systems outside the hospital in the community care system.

The Community System

Conflict

Mary Hogarth (continued from above)

The decision to discharge Ms. Hogarth for noncompliance with treatment forces Dr. Lincoln to set up his patient's aftercare plan more quickly than he would have liked. He finds that Ms. Hogarth has a "case manager," whose role is to coordinate aftercare, and gives her a call:

> DR. LINCOLN [*under pressure*]: Are you Mary Hogarth's case manager? I'm Dr. Lincoln, Mary's doctor. We've got a problem; we have to discharge Mary for breaking unit rules. Since you're her case manager, I guess you're the one who is supposed to set up an aftercare plan. She needs an outpatient therapist and medication follow-up, and . . . oh yeah. Can you get her back into that workshop right away?
>
> CASE MANAGER [*feeling the pressure, and annoyed by Dr. Lincoln's brusque manner*]: Hey, wait a minute. What's going on? I didn't know Mary was going to be discharged. We need time to set this up. I don't even know if she can return to workshop—and there's a waiting list in the outpatient clinic.
>
> DR. L. [*frustrated*]: Well, we don't have time. What's the matter over there? If you can't come up with a plan, we'll just have to discharge her to your office.
>
> CASE MANAGER: That's ridiculous, but if that's how you're going to handle it, there's nothing I can do.

The case manager hangs up angrily, thinking, "Where do these residents get the idea they can push everyone around?" Dr. Lincoln, meanwhile, is enraged, but feels powerless to arrange services for Ms. Hogarth. War has been declared, and Mary Hogarth is caught in no man's land.

Unfortunately, battles like this are all too common when beginning clinicians try to engage the community care system. Dr. Lincoln's anxiety about providing care for Ms. Hogarth quickly, and his lack of information about how to gain access to system resources, have led him to approach the case manager in an insensitive manner that has precipitated increased resistance to his not-unreasonable requests.

Collaboration

As with the ward system, the key to success for Dr. Lincoln in engaging the community system is to avoid an adversarial stance. One way to start is to recognize that Ms. Hogarth's precipitous release places unexpected demands on the system. Because the purpose of her discharge is to accommodate the needs of the ward, not the needs of Ms. Hogarth or her case manager, it would be appropriate for Dr. Lincoln's tone to be apologetic and conciliatory rather than insistent, as in the following interchange:

DR. LINCOLN [*on the phone to Ms. Hogarth's case manager*]: Hi, I'm Dr. Lincoln, Mary Hogarth's doctor on the inpatient unit. I'm sorry that we haven't had a chance to meet yet, but I understand you've been Mary's case manager for a while.

CASE MANAGER: Yes. About 2 years.

DR. L. [*in a friendly manner*]: I bet it hasn't been easy.

CASE MANAGER [*laughing*]: You can say that again.

DR. L.: Well, unfortunately, the reason I called isn't going to make it any easier. We need to discharge Mary from the unit—as soon as possible.

CASE MANAGER [*surprised*]: Why?

DR. L.: I'm sorry we didn't have a chance to discuss this with you sooner, but Mary's been refusing to attend any groups, even though she's close to baseline. It's disrupting the whole unit.

CASE MANAGER: Well, this is par for the course for her; she always has struggled with everyone. The workshop has about had it with her. Anyway, when is she being discharged?

DR. L.: If it were up to the nursing staff it would be this afternoon, but I think we can buy some time to set up a plan. Can you come to the unit this afternoon so we can plan it out?

CASE MANAGER: Well, I'll have to rearrange some things . . . but . . . O.K. I really appreciate that you're trying to be helpful. Some of your fellow residents just call up and scream when they want something done.

In this scenario, Dr. Lincoln is successful in engaging Mary's case manager in a positive relationship in spite of the difficult situation.

Some of the specific techniques that can be employed by the resident are outlined in Table 4–1. The application of these principles is illustrated by the case of Matthew Jermyn, who is being referred by Dr. Transome to a day treatment program.

Table 4–1. Techniques for engaging community caregivers

Engage caregivers as people, not just as "job functions."
Empathize with the caregiver's viewpoint and validate his or her difficulties.
Make no demands, only requests.
Be prepared to extend yourself as much as you would like other caregivers to extend themselves.
Be prepared to offer a next step that can be agreed upon and carried out (e.g., by setting up a meeting or an evaluation).

Matthew Jermyn (continued from p. 58)

Dr. Transome thinks that Mr. Jermyn is ready for referral to the community mental health center's day treatment program. Having visited the program briefly, Dr. Transome thinks it is appropriate, although he is not sure that Mr. Jermyn will fit in.

Because Mr. Jermyn has not always complied with group attendance, Dr. Transome wants to assess the program's level of tolerance and receptivity so that the patient will not be set up to fail. He therefore calls the program director, whom he had previously met, and says that he has a patient who might be a candidate for day treatment, and that he wants the director's opinion. The director, pleased with the resident's interest, agrees to evaluate Mr. Jermyn, although he is skeptical about the patient's chances.

Dr. Transome offers to come along to see what the program is like from the perspective of a patient, as well as to help Mr. Jermyn make the transition from his care. Mr. Jermyn is accepted, but even if he had not been, Dr. Transome's time has been well spent. He now has a better feel for how the day program works, which will help with future referrals, and he has earned the good will of the day treatment staff.

The more residents know about the agencies, services, and staff in their own care system, the more effective they will be in engaging the system successfully to meet the needs of their patients. We will discuss this process in more detail in the next section.

Engaging and Assessing the Community System

A community mental health clinic in a Boston suburb routinely orients all incoming staff and trainees with a community tour conducted by senior staff. This tour usually takes 1 or 2 days and includes visits to all the significant program sites in the community, with introductions to key staff and a review of each agency's program. The key information is included in a comprehensive resource directory.

If a residency does not provide such a tour, residents can organize it on their own. In any case, they can collect pertinent data about the programs in their community and put them together in a personal resource manual. The *community system assessment protocol* (see Appendix C) can be used as an outline for such a manual; it illustrates some of the questions clinicians might ask to assess resources and programs. The following issues are particularly important.

Level of case management responsibility. Some programs assume full responsibility for case management in the context of an integrated and comprehensive service delivery system. More commonly, however, case managers broker services with individual programs that assume responsibility only for the portion of the client's life that is covered by that program. Whenever a resident sets up programs for a client, therefore, the question of who has overall case management responsibility must be answered. Because in most systems this role is not clearly defined, residents need to assess their own responsibilities for coordination and administration.

The role of the therapist or medicating physician is in some ways similar to that of case manager. While the case manager is hired to broker services and transport clients to appointments, it is sometimes not clear who decides what services are needed and when. The case manager may assume responsibility for this clinical leadership function by default unless the resident or other primary clinician is prepared to take it on.

Accessibility of emergency services and hospitalization. In Chapters 2 and 3, ensuring safety for patient, family, and clinician was discussed as a necessary precondition for successful engagement in a treatment relationship. An important aspect of ensuring safety is ready access to a 24-hour emergency service and to hospitalization. If a resident determines that emergency intervention and/or hospitalization are necessary, but he or she is powerless to arrange for emergency admission, both the resident and the patient will feel unsafe. Residents therefore need to learn the means of access to these services before an emergency actually occurs. Building positive relationships with key "gatekeepers" is the best strategy to facilitate this process.

Assessment of requirements for participation. Simply helping a patient to gain admission to a program does not complete the resident's task. Residents also need to try to predict whether patients can remain in a program, as in the following example, by assessing whether they can meet the specific requirements for participation:

> Alice Jenkins, a 21-year old woman with schizophrenia, enters a community residence. She willingly attends day treatment, but refuses to take her prescribed medication. Because the residence at first takes the position that it has no right to force the patient to take medication, the patient decompensates and is rehospitalized.

Engagement of self-help programs. Starting in the 1980s, there has been rapid growth in self-help programs of support for mentally ill persons (e.g., Recovery, Inc.; Schizophrenics Anonymous; Manic-Depressive Association); for addicted individuals (e.g., Alcoholics

Anonymous, Narcotics Anonymous, Cocaine Anonymous); and for the families of both groups (e.g., Alliance for the Mentally Ill, Alanon, Naranon). Although only a few of these programs have a distinctly antipsychiatric focus (e.g., Mental Patients' Liberation Front), they all caution patients and their families to beware of the shortcomings of the professional community and to rely on peer support to overcome these shortcomings. Residents and other beginning clinicians may feel uncomfortable with the way these programs challenge their professional competence and, therefore, may avoid finding out how they really work.

If, however, residents engage with self-help programs, they will usually discover a great potential source of support for their patients and their patients' families, and a possible addition to their therapeutic arsenal. Although one can learn about these programs by reading their literature, the best way to learn about them is to attend meetings to see how they operate. To get the most from a visit, residents need to let their professional guard down; to be as open, receptive, and conciliatory as possible; and to maintain an attitude of trying to understand why the programs work, rather than trying to prove that they do not. (Self-help programs in substance abuse treatment for mentally ill patients with such problems will be discussed further in Chapter 10.)

Assessment of generic services. Not all needed services for mentally ill individuals must be provided within the mental health service system; for example, the local social services department may be the agency that provides financial assistance for a patient. All community services in one way or another may provide assistance to the mentally ill person and so need to be included in an assessment of available community support.

Gaps in the system. The eligibility, participation requirements, and other characteristics of a community's programs inevitably leave gaps, so that some of the services needed for some patients will be unavailable. These gaps in resources define the "cracks" in the system. In order to analyze the system as a whole, therefore, the resident needs to understand what happens to patients who fall through the cracks. Some of the specific questions that have answers which indicate where these gaps occur—and, therefore, when it may be particularly difficult to arrange for aftercare for a specific patient—are provided in Table 4–2.

Before demonstrating how the community system works, we will discuss the assessment of one more system, the legal system.

Table 4–2. Assessing the cracks in the community system

1. What happens to patients who have no place to live?
   a. Are patients discharged to the streets?
   b. If so, under what circumstances, and what programs are available for such patients?
   c. Under what circumstances can patients be hospitalized—or remain hospitalized—in order to be placed in an appropriate residence?
   d. What are the waiting lists like for different types of residence programs? How are the lists prioritized, and where do patients wait?
   e. Are respite programs and other crisis residential alternatives available?

2. What happens to patients who have no treatment?
   a. Are patients discharged without case management? without psychiatric treatment? without therapists? without day treatment or rehabilitation?
   b. What are the waiting lists like for each type of service?
   c. What programs are available to provide support to patients who are waiting (e.g., 24-hour crisis services, emergency psychiatric care, holding groups, drop-in centers, clubhouses)?

3. What happens to patients who have no money?
   a. What are the limitations of available welfare payments and food stamps for patients with or without SSI/SSDI?
   b. What sources of emergency funds, rental subsidies, food assistance (e.g., soup kitchens, food stamps) are available?
   c. What is the waiting period for disability benefits?
   d. What does Medicaid provide in each category, and what medical services are available to those patients with no coverage?
   e. Is there a source of free medication?

Engaging and Assessing the Legal System

Dale Wharton (continued from p. 53)

After Dale Wharton is admitted to the open unit for threatening his parents (Chapter 3), he begins to refuse medication. Dr. Lincoln meets with Mr. Wharton to assess the situation:

> DR. LINCOLN: I understand you've been refusing your medication. Could you tell me about what's going on?

MR. WHARTON: Look, I don't want to be here—it's my parents' idea—so I won't take your damn pills. They're poison, anyway.

DR. L.: Does the medicine help in any way?

MR. W.: Sure—it helps you goddam doctors run my life. It does me no damn good.

DR. L.: So why did you take it at home?

MR. W.: Who says I did? Anyway, I only took it once in a while—just to get my parents off my back.

Dr. Lincoln leaves the room feeling anxious and uncertain. He can understand why Mr. Wharton's parents think their son is dangerous; he also felt frightened during Mr. Wharton's last outburst. But he is not sure whether it is safe for his patient to remain on the open unit; if not, can he be committed to a locked unit? And does he, Dr. Lincoln, have the power—or the right—to force him to take medicine?

On the one hand, Dr. Lincoln knows that without medication, Mr. Wharton will only get worse; on the other hand, his patient is not totally irrational—and seems to be aware of the dangers of neuroleptics—so Dr. Lincoln feels uncomfortable about taking away the patient's right to refuse treatment.

As this case illustrates, Dr. Lincoln needs to be familiar with the mental health legal system in order for him to enforce treatment or ensure medication compliance. The legal issues are often not clear-cut, and residents understandably prefer to focus on diagnosis and treatment. Yet, paradoxically, the more comfortable that residents feel with the exercise of their legal power—and the more clearly they know its limits—the more likely it is that their patients' treatment will proceed smoothly. Unfortunately, each jurisdiction has its own laws; a series of questions covering the areas with which residents need to become familiar are provided in Appendix D.

As yet, Dr. Lincoln has not become familiar with the legal issues in his state, so he consults his supervisor, who reviews the legal issues in Mr. Wharton's case and observes the following:

First, Mr. Wharton is indeed committable, because he had been violent toward his parents and was threatening toward Dr. Lincoln. Mr. Wharton's angry outbursts and treatment refusal make it likely that he will need a secure unit.

Second, Mr. Wharton is a probable candidate for medication guardianship. Even though he is aware of the risks of medication, he cannot accurately assess its benefits because of his denial. He reveals auditory hallucinations, but has no insight that these are symptoms of illness rather than real voices. A patient who is clearly mentally ill but does not believe he is ill is likely to be considered incompetent to make medication decisions, and therefore could be given medication involuntarily.

The supervisor also points out that even though Dr. Lincoln potentially has the legal power to enforce treatment, it would be better if Mr. Wharton could be engaged to accept treatment voluntarily. Consequently, the supervisor suggests that Dr. Lincoln offer Mr. Wharton a choice of medication compliance or involuntary commitment (with medication guardianship). When Dr. Lincoln offers this choice, Mr. Wharton does not back down. Dr. Lincoln gives him 2 days to think it over, but Mr. Wharton becomes more paranoid, loose, and threatening and continues to refuse medication, and is thus committed to the locked unit under the care of Dr. Smythe:

MR. WHARTON: I won't take medication.

DR. SMYTHE: Why not?

MR. W.: There's nothing wrong with me. God told me I'm fine. He tells me to get rid of evil and I will obey.

DR. S. [*observing that Mr. Wharton's denial of his psychotic illness is so severe that he is not competent to make rational decisions about medication*]: I would like you to take medication voluntarily, but if you won't we will begin the process to give it to you involuntarily. It's your choice.

MR. W.: God will set me free. No meds! No meds!

DR. S. [*calmly*]: O.K. We'll make sure you get the help you need even if you're not able to accept it.

Dr. Smythe's familiarity with his state's legal system prevents an unnecessary struggle; he simply initiates the legal process to administer medication involuntarily.

Initially, it may be frightening for residents to deal with lawyers and judges, to appear as witnesses, to sign depositions, or to be subject to cross-examination. However, the principles of teamwork and engagement apply to the legal system as well as to the ward and community systems, and although the legal system is an adversarial system, it is often possible to avoid an adversarial stance.

Suppose Mr. Wharton has a court-appointed attorney present in his hearing about receiving involuntary medication. If Dr. Smythe assumes that the attorney is his enemy, he is likely to feel angry at being challenged or questioned. If, however, he assumes from the beginning that the attorney is concerned with the client's best interests and is legitimately present to protect the client's rights, he will find it easier to work with the attorney and the legal system in a joint effort to do what is best for Mr. Wharton. Even though the attorney's priorities and the psychiatrist's priorities may differ, these participants can still collaborate in an atmosphere of mutual respect. (For a more comprehensive discussion of the psychiatrist's relationship with the law and lawyers, see GAP Report No. 131, *The Mental Health Professional and the Legal System.*)

We next turn to the application of the principles of systems assessment to the psychosocial evaluation of an individual case.

Assessing the Patient's System of Care

As we noted in Chapters 2 and 3, the biopsychosocial assessment protocol (see Appendix A) provides a model for assessment of the patient's involvement with the care system and with his or her environment in general.

Collecting Data

The resident should ask the patient, the family, and all involved caregivers about the patient's current and past involvement with each community system. Significant past caregivers may also be contacted, particularly when there is confusion about the history.

Generally, different caregivers from different programs will see the patient and family differently. Variations in how the patient is perceived in different settings provide important data for placement decisions.

System stereotypes, such as "She's just a borderline," "He can't succeed at day treatment," or "This family can't be engaged," often become generalized as permanent characteristics of the patient or family that predict repeated failure and therefore can stifle further therapeutic effort. Critically reviewing the data that support these stereotypes may show that the stereotypes are unfounded and that more positive formulations are possible.

Note that the patient, family, and caregivers may disagree. For example, a patient's main problem, according to his or her case manager, may be that he or she "needs a residential placement, but no placement is available." The patient, on the other hand, may not want a placement, and the family may be ambivalent, so even if a placement were available, the patient would probably refuse it. Thus, the "main problem" is that the patient needs services but is not yet ready to accept them.

Performing Multidimensional Longitudinal Assessment

In Matthew Jermyn's case (see Chapter 2), the loss of a therapist contributed to the patient's medication noncompliance and poor level of functioning over a period of years. Thus, an important function of the longitudinal systems assessment is to ascertain the optimal pace of progress through the system. Success is often the chronic patient's worst enemy: patients who take a small step ahead may then try to race forward into "health," and instead wind up with a full-blown relapse, as in the following example:

> David Booth, a 20-year-old man with schizophrenia and significant denial, had nonetheless done well in a community residence and day program for 3 years. When the patient began a part-time job, however, he performed more poorly than he had expected. He incorrectly attributed this to a medication side effect, began refusing medication, and after 4 months became psychotic and had to be rehospitalized. Meanwhile, his psychotic behavior was so disturbing that he lost his residential placement. The relationship of his behavior to the job placement and subsequent medication refusal, overlooked by the residential program, was not picked up until the inpatient psychiatry resident did a thorough systems assessment.

As this case indicates, data from the "systems" assessment need to be placed in chronological sequence on a time line and fit together with data from the assessments of the illness, the individual, and the family.

This comprehensive assessment format can be applied to the case of Mary Hogarth:

Mary Hogarth (continued from p. 63)

> As noted earlier, Dr. Lincoln and Ms. Hogarth's case manager agreed to meet to set up a discharge plan for her. The first task of the meeting, however, is to complete Ms. Hogarth's assessment and to develop a formulation to identify her future treatment and case management needs. Dr. Lincoln has spoken to Ms. Hogarth, to her mother, and to the director of Ms. Hogarth's workshop. The case manager over 2 years has gathered considerable data about Ms. Hogarth's systems history and shares this information with Dr. Lincoln. The following picture emerges:
>
>> Ms. Hogarth, the only child of her widowed mother, had been hospitalized for the first time 5 years before with a severe psychotic decompensation. At the time, she was working as a hotel maid and living at home. She had never dated and had few social contacts. Her adjustment at best could be characterized as schizoid; at worst she may have been chronically disorganized for years prior to her first overt "break."

The immediate precipitant of Ms. Hogarth's psychosis was an episode in which a hotel guest had attempted to seduce her. She became panicky and developed delusions about being followed, attacked, and torn apart, along with accusatory voices calling her a "slut" and a "whore." Following hospitalization, she continued to hear voices and never regained her original baseline.

Her mother, who is alone in the world except for her daughter, has never accepted the seriousness of her daughter's illness. The mother feels that it was the medicine that caused her daughter's regression, and encourages her to skip doses when she is having a bad day. Ms. Hogarth's mother also feels that most treatment programs do not understand her daughter's needs and "make her sicker."

Ms. Hogarth and her mother have resisted any engagement in "talking therapy," preferring to seek support in their own church. Ms. Hogarth attends only medication clinic, and that intermittently. Aggressive outreach by a succession of frustrated case managers has managed to keep her on enough medicine to prevent relapse, but her mental status has fluctuated widely under stress.

Day treatment and social rehabilitation programs had been unsuccessful. Ms. Hogarth found unstructured social interaction, especially with men, to be frightening and to lead to increased symptoms, the same dynamic which kept her from participating in groups on the ward. Attempts to return to competitive work settings were also overwhelming. For the past year, however, Mary has participated in a sheltered workshop and, for the first time, seems engaged. Repetitive work and limited social involvement are organizing factors for her, and her mother feels more comfortable with a vocational rather than a therapeutic focus. Most important, the director of the workshop at the time Mary started the program was a maternal figure with whom Mary rapidly developed rapport.

Unfortunately, 3 months prior to the present admission, the workshop director left and was replaced by a younger woman whom Mary did not like as well. Also, one of the retarded men at the program began flirting with her. Ms. Hogarth began skipping her medicine more often; her workshop attendance decreased, and visits to the emergency room with "anxiety" became more frequent. On the day of admission, the man at the program tried to kiss her, and she immediately decompensated.

Staff at the workshop like Ms. Hogarth, who can be quite pleasant when compensated, but are beginning to feel fed up with her. All of her caregivers feel that residential placement might be helpful, but the patient and her mother are adamantly opposed. Medication guardianship has also been proposed—and rejected.

Ms. Hogarth would have to go home after discharge. Her ability to attend the workshop was questionable, although she said she wanted to go. Her mother thought she needed a new program, but where? And what about medication compliance?

In discussing the assessment, Dr. Lincoln and the case manager see clearly the interaction between Ms. Hogarth's illness, her individual and family dynamics, and her successes and failures in community placement. They extend their empathy not only to Ms. Hogarth and her mother, but to the caregivers at the workshop who have tried so hard to work with her. The anger they feel at Ms. Hogarth for getting herself discharged has softened, but they still feel frustrated. The issues are now clear, but the plan is not.

5

Developing and Implementing a Treatment Plan

The next step after completing the assessment of a patient is the challenging task of developing a treatment plan. In this chapter, we attempt to provide some general guidelines and priorities to help structure the treatment planning process. The treatment plan is ideally a kind of "road map," providing a structured expression of treatment priorities, beginning with the most pressing immediate concerns and leading, in sequence, to the stabilization and rehabilitation of the patient. In ordering these priorities, the resident needs to define clearly the problems confronting the patient and then to set immediate, short-term, and long-term goals.

Guidelines for Setting Priorities in Treatment Planning

Although treatment planning inevitably includes trial and error, it is not completely random. While the issues often overlap and many of them must be addressed simultaneously, setting priorities helps to organize strategic thinking and may be crucial to decision making.

A Case Example

The following case example of a chronically psychotic patient demonstrates the development and application of priorities to planning treatment and implementing the plan:

Thomas Maddox[1]

Thomas Maddox, a 30-year-old man with a long-standing diagnosis of schizophrenia, was recently discharged from the hospital and has just been assigned to Dr. Wilcox in an outpatient clinic. Mr. Maddox's psychotic symptoms, which began in his first year of college, have required hospitalization on about a dozen occasions, usually after the patient stops taking his medication. He describes himself as a "nervous person" who takes medicine to "calm down." He is currently medication compliant, but says the medicine "isn't working very well." He is also unable to recognize the impact of illness on his life, on his ability to complete college, and on his social isolation. When asked about past losses and future goals, he becomes anxious and says he does not want to discuss these topics.

Despite his current medication compliance, Mr. Maddox continues to have significant psychotic symptoms, including persistent paranoia, violent fantasies, and bothersome intrusive thoughts. In recent years his level of baseline functioning has deteriorated, and he has needed higher doses of medication to maintain stability. As a result, he reports more side effects, particularly restless legs.

Mr. Maddox's parents have been disappointed in past treatment efforts and have often felt excluded from participation in treatment. While Mrs. Maddox is fairly tolerant of her son's poor performance, her husband is more critical. He is concerned about his son's difficulty in showering and his pattern of sleeping for 2 days and then remaining awake for 2 days. He attributes the sleep pattern to all the caffeine his son consumes, but he has not been able to convince his son to stop drinking so much coffee. He also worries about his son's staying home all day and wishes he would get out and "do something."

In the past Mr. Maddox had been assigned to a clinic medication group. Because he suffered from paranoid ideas about the other group members, his alliance with the group leaders was tentative, his attendance at group meetings was sporadic, and his medication compliance was poor.

---

[1]In the illustration, the resident, Dr. Wilcox, is able to treat his patient over 3 years; it is not always possible, however, for residents to follow patients over such a long time, and compromises often have to be made, usually by transferring patients to other residents. But no matter how carefully patients and residents are prepared for such transfers, these vulnerable patients are likely to regress at least to some degree. Whenever possible, therefore, such transfers should be avoided; if it is not possible to avoid them, a transitional period in which both residents work together with patient and family can help to reduce the extent of the regression.

> Mr. Maddox and his parents believe that friendly personal care would be more helpful than intensive individual or group therapy, and the patient is opposed to day treatment. He complains that the medication makes him restless and uncomfortable rather than "calm," and he admits to many bothersome thoughts. He agrees to see Dr. Wilcox occasionally for help with these problems.

Based on the information gathered in the initial session, Dr. Wilcox concludes that 1) Mr. Maddox suffers from chronic paranoid schizophrenia with acute exacerbations about once a year, caused primarily by discontinuation of medication; 2) the patient has significant akathisia, which seems to have contributed to the difficulty in compliance; and 3) although the family is interested, involved, and supportive, it is also confused, divided, and in need of guidance as well as more direct involvement with the psychiatrist. Dr. Wilcox thinks that although Mr. Maddox might eventually benefit from intensive day treatment and social rehabilitation, the patient is at present much too resistant and paranoid even to consider such a plan.

After discussing the situation with his supervisor, Dr. Wilcox sets planning and treatment priorities as defined in Chapter 2, and as outlined in Table 5–1.

Maintaining safety and containment. Dr. Wilcox talks with Mr. Maddox and his family about whether he could manage safely at home or needs to be in the hospital. The family says that he is eating well and not engaging in dangerous activities at home. The patient denies suicidal or homicidal thoughts, and, although he is vaguely paranoid about his parents, he denies command hallucinations. Both the family and the patient conclude that they are willing to continue outpatient treatment. Dr. Wilcox discusses what would be strong indicators for rehospitalization, such as suicidal thoughts, dangerous behavior, refusal to eat, severe agitation, and so forth, and the parents agree to notify Dr. Wilcox if any of these indicators appear.

Establishing and protecting the therapeutic alliance. Dr. Wilcox decides that as the medicating psychiatrist, he has the best chance of engaging the Maddoxes, as they are so skeptical about any psychological approach. Even so, establishing a stable and effective therapeutic alliance with the patient has proved difficult. The patient's determination to avoid medication side effects makes him resist proposed medication changes, and he is reluctant to trust yet another in a series of psychiatrists.

By having regular meetings with Mr. Maddox's parents as well as with Mr. Maddox, Dr. Wilcox hopes to relate quickly to the parents. This alliance,

Table 5–1. Treatment plan for Thomas Maddox (see text for background)

A. Immediate goals

1. Maintain safety and containment.
   a. Assess the patient for dangerousness to self or others.
   b. Review patient's behavior with family members.
   c. Establish collaborative plan for notification of clinician if patient's behavior deteriorates or family members become concerned.

B. Short-term goals

1. Establish and protect the therapeutic alliance.
   a. Meet regularly with both patient and parents.
      i. With parents, focus on support; educate regarding residual and prodromal symptoms.
      ii. With patient, explore concerns about medication, particularly about side effects; educate about the function of medication and the risks of relapse.
2. Control acute symptoms.
   a. Adjust medication to obtain optimal symptom control and the least number and severity of side effects.
   b. Consider depot medication.

C. Intermediate-term goals

1. Maintain stability throughout convalescence.
   a. Begin to mobilize the patient.
      i. Create a daily structure involving patient's maintenance of personal hygiene and use of graded tasks and expectations.
      ii. Deal with loneliness by a) initiating and helping patient perform structured but undemanding social activities; and b) helping patient to begin work on social skills.

D. Long-term goals

1. Monitor and assist rehabilitation and growth.
   a. Help patient adjust to sheltered work setting.
   b. Provide active social skills training.
   c. Initiate more intensive psychotherapy.
   d. Explore potential for additional progress.

by supplementing the tenuous initial connection with the patient, will permit him to begin to work on the task of controlling symptoms.

A more effective, trusting relationship with the patient in this case took many months to establish. Only after prolonged and patient effort could Mr. Maddox gradually begin to open up and describe his illness experience. Eventually, this dialogue made it possible for Dr. Wilcox to begin to educate the patient about his illness.

Meanwhile, Dr. Wilcox is able to use the patient's parents' need for support, education, and guidance to involve them more closely. As one outcome of this involvement, the patient's father has begun to recognize that Mr. Maddox's passivity is not merely a matter of laziness and that his son will not respond simply to pressure.

Controlling acute symptoms. Once a beginning alliance is established, Dr. Wilcox proposes and the patient accepts a medication change designed to alleviate some of Mr. Maddox's akathisia. Dr. Wilcox hopes that this change will make the patient more comfortable and more medication compliant, which would in turn strengthen the therapeutic alliance with both the patient and his family.[2]

As their relationship progresses, Mr. Maddox becomes more comfortable with Dr. Wilcox and develops greater trust in him; because he feels accepted by Dr. Wilcox, he can now turn to him for advice. Finally, after considerable discussion, Mr. Maddox agrees that a change in medication to a long-acting depot-type drug might make him less reluctant to take medication. Over the next year, with depot medication, his residual psychotic symptoms gradually recede.

Maintaining stability through convalescence. Mr. Maddox eventually agrees that it would be easier to maintain stability if he felt less lonely and bored, and more comfortable with other people. With much support and encouragement he agrees to attend a drop-in day treatment center. After some adjustment difficulties, he does well with this treatment program.

A year later his father suggests, with increasing urgency, that it is time for his son to begin working. He insists that his son is "stagnating" in the day program and thinks that his clinicians are "too timid and conservative." Mr. Maddox seems all too willing to believe that he no

---

[2]In setting his initial treatment priorities, Dr. Wilcox had decided that it would be counterproductive to press the patient for medication changes before an effective alliance was established with both the patient and his parents, so that effective symptom control was established only after the alliances were reasonably strong.

longer needs careful monitoring and seems to want very much to please his father. It is only after he begins to exhibit recurrent psychotic symptoms and to insist he no longer needs his Prolixin shot that it is possible to persuade both patient and family to adopt a more realistic pace.

Facilitating rehabilitation and growth. In meetings with the Maddox family, a daily structure is established for their son and gradually implemented. First, the structure is limited to improving the patient's personal hygiene and decreasing his caffeine intake. Although he reluctantly complies, Mr. Maddox is often uncomfortable with the effort involved and at first is not at all convinced that these activities will lead to a useful result. He becomes more convinced as his symptoms continue to be in good control and as he is less troubled by side effects.

Mr. Maddox improves gradually and steadily. His appointments with Dr. Wilcox initially included his parents, but in the third year of treatment, as he feels less fearful and more comfortable, he asks for individual sessions. Together, Dr. Wilcox and Mr. Maddox conclude that he is ready to take on some new challenges, and they discuss longer-term goals. Mr. Maddox begins to consider the possibility of getting a job and enrolls in a state rehabilitation program. He also attends a social skills training group after he expresses a wish to feel more at ease with people his own age. Because family issues are no longer pressing, the family sessions are decreased to once per month. Eventually, Mr. Maddox is able to work at a low-stress job, to take some night school courses, and to establish gradually a limited but rewarding social life.

Further Examples of Setting Treatment Guidelines

Many of Mr. Jermyn's treatment issues are similar to those of Mr. Maddox:

Matthew Jermyn *(continued from p. 65)*

Alliance: In the hospital Dr. Transome succeeds in developing rapport with both Mr. Jermyn and his parents, and can then cement the alliance by setting up regular follow-up meetings, alternating time with the patient and with the family.

Symptom control and maintenance: Using the support of these meetings, Mr. Jermyn's parents gradually become able to require their son to maintain medication compliance on intramuscular (IM) meds as a condition of living at home. Mr. Jermyn confides to Dr. Transome that he is relieved that he will not be able to decide to stop his meds.

Growth and rehabilitation: Mr. Jermyn finally enters a period of prolonged stability and convalescence. In his individual work with Dr. Transome, he slowly starts to address his painful feelings of loss and loneliness, which leads eventually to his willingness to participate in a vocational clubhouse program and to begin to reconnect with society.

Ms. DeBarry (continued from p. 8)

The first concern of Dr. Lyon is for Ms. DeBarry's safety. After unsuccessfully struggling through several chaotic weeks of attempted treatment, Dr. Lyon, with the support of his supervisor, insists that Ms. DeBarry enter the hospital voluntarily as a precondition for continued outpatient treatment. To Dr. Lyon's surprise, Ms. DeBarry complies readily when she realizes that her therapist will not back down.

Alliance: Dr. Lyon is finally able to begin to establish rapport with Ms. DeBarry. The patient's mother acknowledges that she too has been frustrated by Ms. DeBarry's erratic behavior. Dr. Lyon suggests to the mother that they meet periodically to compare notes and prevent miscommunication; the mother, feeling supported, readily agrees.

Acute control of symptoms: In the hospital, Ms. DeBarry's affective symptoms are regulated satisfactorily with a combination of lithium and valproic acid.

Maintenance and convalescence: Dr. Lyon's discharge plan provides structure and limits to encourage compliance and stability. It includes weekly individual psychotherapy meetings; weekly prescriptions and, initially, weekly blood levels; weekly phone contact and monthly meetings with Ms. DeBarry's mother; and a contract for rehospitalization in the event of medication noncompliance, suicidal threats/behavior, or repeated failure to keep appointments. Day treatment is also proposed, but rejected. Dr. Lyon feels he has no leverage to insist on this point at this time, but notes to the patient and her mother that if the current plan does not work, additional structure may be required in the future.

Growth and rehabilitation: Dr. Lyon's long-term goal is to stabilize Ms. DeBarry with medication and structure, and to help her discuss her feelings with him in therapy rather than act them out. Once her behavior becomes more consistent, Dr. Lyon will consider a referral for vocational rehabilitation or supported employment.

Mary Hogarth (continued from p. 74)

Dr. Lincoln and the case manager focus first on how to develop an alliance with Ms. Hogarth and her mother. In the Hogarths' case, it seems that regular home visits by the case manager are the intervention that is most likely to help the mother to engage. Dr. Lincoln volunteers to accompany the case manager on the first home visit in order to reinforce the importance of medication compliance.

Maintaining control of symptoms: Symptoms may be controlled by making Ms. Hogarth's return to the workshop conditional on beginning depot medication in the hospital. At a joint meeting, Ms. Hogarth's mother is pleased with the idea of home visits, but uncertain about depot medication, and worries about her daughter's returning to the same workshop. Dr. Lincoln suggests that with a shot, Ms. Hogarth would probably need less medication and would be able to work more consistently. He also proposes that Ms. Hogarth should not go back to the workshop immediately, but instead remain at home "convalescing" for a few weeks while her new medication is being regulated. During this time, the case manager would attempt to negotiate with the workshop to transfer Ms. Hogarth to a different work site, as well as arrange for the visiting nurse to administer her medication at the workshop. One of the senior female counselors at the workshop would work with Ms. Hogarth as a supportive contact person to help compensate for the loss of the workshop director.

Rehabilitation and growth: Both Ms. Hogarth and her mother are willing to accept this short-term plan. Dr. Lincoln and the case manager recognize that eventually Ms. Hogarth will need to develop improved skills for independence, for socialization, and for dealing with feelings of loss, loneliness, and fear of sexual assault. Similarly, Ms. Hogarth's mother needs to improve her understanding of her daughter's illness and her need for medication. Although none of these long-term goals can be addressed immediately, they could be explored by the case manager and by workshop staff when Ms. Hogarth and her mother have been successfully engaged and the patient stabilized. Perhaps in 1 to 2 years, a referral for individual and/or family therapy could be made. The possibility of eventual residential placement is even farther in the future.

6

The Art of Prescribing Medication

Matthew Jermyn (continued from p. 81)

In developing a treatment plan for Mr. Jermyn (see Chapters 3 and 5), Dr. Transome had worked out a contract with Mr. Jermyn's parents in which the Jermyns agreed to allow their son home only on condition that he take intramuscularly administered fluphenazine regularly. Mr. Jermyn was initially resistant, but when he saw that his parents were serious, he went along. Mr. Jermyn began his intramuscular (im) medication in the hospital to adjust the dosage, and then continued to receive shots every 2 weeks after discharge. The shots were given by Dr. Transome in his office following brief individual therapy sessions.

Approximately 3 months after discharge from the hospital, Mr. Jermyn announces to Dr. Transome that he no longer wants his shot. He says that it makes him "too sleepy to work," although he is clearly still disoriented. He agrees to take some pills "if I need them," but says, "I'm not really sick any more, you know, and those medicines dull my brain."

Dr. Transome phones the Jermyns, who are not surprised. "He's been acting up lately," says Mr. Jermyn's father. "I figured something was brewing. He always stops medicine about now." "Maybe he's on too much," adds his mother. "He does sleep a lot now, and he eats all the time." They both express considerable ambivalence about enforcing their contract, even though they know their son will soon get sick again. "We can't just kick him out, he *is* our son."

Dr. Transome is frustrated. All his plans to keep Mr. Jermyn on medicine seem to be falling apart. He recognizes that without ongoing medication compliance, all other therapeutic and rehabilitative efforts are unlikely to succeed.

Consequently, Dr. Transome needs to develop a strategy for controlling acute symptoms by maintaining Mr. Jermyn's medication compliance. Unfortunately, despite the clear importance of ongoing medication, both patients and families will often exhibit surprising—and frustrating—resistances to the resident's efforts to promote compliance. There are many reasons for this resistance, which are discussed below.

Reasons for Resistance to Medication Compliance

Denial

Denial of illness. Even when adequately medicated, many chronically mentally ill patients persist in denying their mental illness, viewing medication as an unjustified chemical invasion of their bodies by the psychiatrist, often with the "collusion" of their families. Patients whose psychoses completely clear when on medication may minimize or even totally repress their recollection of the psychosis that necessitated medication in the first place. For these patients, accepting the need for medication may be associated with painful feelings of stigma and narcissistic injury related to acknowledging the mental illness. Residents may find that such feelings can also lead family members to exhibit surprisingly profound denial and to support, overtly or covertly, the patient's resistance to medication maintenance.

Avoidance of reality. For many patients, the success of medication in eliminating psychotic symptoms brings them face to face with the dismal reality of their lives. Rather than face the pain and dysphoria associated with acknowledging illness and disability, patients may discontinue medications to bring back grandiose psychotic ideas associated with euphoria and denial of unpleasant reality.

Denial of chronicity. A common source of resistance to taking antipsychotic medication for prophylaxis against relapse is the fact that doing so implies that the patient suffers from a chronic, recurrent illness in which the risk of relapse continues indefinitely. Understandably, most patients and families find this a difficult idea to accept. As a result, they often are determined to demonstrate that they can avoid psychosis without the aid of medication.

Patients and families often do not recognize that medication is used both to control acute symptoms and to prevent relapse. Usually, patients are stabilized on a relatively high dose of medication, which is gradually reduced to a "maintenance level." As patients improve, however, they and their families may regard the medication only as a sedative or "tranquilizer"; therefore, once the patients' symptoms have subsided, they are viewed as "back to normal," and the "tranquilizer" is considered to be no longer required.

Medication Effects

Discomfort due to side effects. Some patients object strongly to the subjective experience of being medicated. Their objection may be related to unpleasant side effects, sedation, dystonia, or akathisia, or it may result from the primary effect of the drug—a subjective sense of being psychologically changed in ways that are disconcerting and unpleasant. Patients who do not believe that they need medication will focus on even minor side effects as an excuse to discontinue the medication; even if they are aware that the medication has been helpful, their subjective discomfort may lead to complaints, opposition to medicine, and medicine refusal.

Families may also object to the medication effects. When, on their early visits to a hospitalized relative on high doses of antipsychotic medication, they see a sedated, rigid, relatively immobile patient who complains of restlessness and blurred vision, they may indignantly question whether the treatment is worse than the illness.

Incomplete medication efficacy. A significant source of medication resistance for many patients and families is the fact that antipsychotic medications frequently do not completely eliminate the symptoms of mental illness. Patients whose positive or negative symptoms persist even when they are adequately medicated understandably feel that the medicine is "doing no good." Often the medicine is then blamed for causing the symptoms, rather than viewed as ameliorating them. Patients and families soon forget or deny how much worse the illness was before the medicine was started. These attitudes readily lead to medication noncompliance.

Fear of tardive dyskinesia. Patient resistance to taking neuroleptic medication on a continuing basis is enhanced by concerns about the long-term risk of tardive dyskinesia (TD). Their concerns are often stirred up during the process of obtaining informed consent for long-term neuroleptic use. Because TD is extremely rare in the first few months of treatment with neuroleptics, the clinician can usually safely defer discussion of TD with the patient until the acute psychotic episode is over, but the risk of TD cannot be ignored indefinitely.

Patients are understandably concerned about this risk, because TD ultimately affects a significant number of patients on chronic maintenance neuroleptic medication. Patients and families may use their concern about TD to reinforce their wish that long-term medication is not necessary and should be discontinued. Moreover, patients, families, and clinicians alike may exaggerate the long-term risk of TD, which is relatively small compared to the near certain immediate risks associated with psychotic relapse following medication discontinuation.

Absence of immediate relapse. Because of the persistent effects of neuroleptics, a patient may not suffer recurrent psychotic symptoms for weeks or even months after discontinuing the medication. In fact, it generally takes 3 to 6 months before relapse occurs in a patient stabilized over a year who discontinues medication. Thus, a patient who questions the need for medication may begin by skipping several doses or reducing the dose; because there is no immediate reappearance of psychotic symptoms, the patient may feel reassured that the clinician was being too conservative and that the medication was not really necessary.

Autonomy Issues

Strivings for independence. Medication noncompliance may result as much from resistance to being compliant as from resistance to taking medication. Many young people who develop mental illness are at a developmental phase in which a certain amount of rebellion is not only expected but healthy. In these people the insistence on ongoing medication compliance by both medical and parental authority figures will naturally engender a wish to rebel; noncompliance may be the only means by which the patient can express his or her strivings to be more independent.

Concerns about forcing medication. The other side of the autonomy issue is the ambivalence that families—and residents—may have about insisting that patients remain medication compliant. As in the case of the Jermyns, parents may be more concerned about upsetting their child or harming him or her with medication side effects than with ensuring his or her only chance at recovery by taking a strong stand on the need for compliance. Patients—like Matthew Jermyn—who find that by loudly resisting medicine they can make their parents—and doctors—back down, often conclude that the medicine is really not crucial, which thereby reinforces their wish to deny their illness.

Resistance to "dependence on tranquilizers." For some patients and families, "dependence on tranquilizers" is viewed as a sign of moral or psychological weakness, and therefore must be avoided at all costs. In such cases, continuing medication may be regarded as a sign of "addiction," which may be considered more serious than the original psychosis. In fact, "health" may be defined more by being "off medicine" than by being symptom free, and the patient's relapse when off medication may only reinforce the perception that he or she is addicted. In some families, patients have even been accused of malingering symptoms to fool the psychiatrist into prescribing medication.

Many of the reasons listed above contributed to Matthew Jermyn's decision to refuse im fluphenazine and to his parents' reluctance to enforce medication compliance as a condition for Matthew's living at home. Like most residents, Dr. Transome is faced with the problem of how to overcome these resistances when they arise. In the remainder of this chapter we will address the development of a coherent strategy for prescribing medication and maintaining medication compliance for chronically mentally ill patients.

Strategies for Medication Compliance

The major elements of a coherent strategy for medicating chronically mentally ill patients (see Table 6–1) are discussed below.

Collaborative Relationship

As in every other aspect of treatment, a trusting, collaborative relationship with the patient and family is essential for successful long-term treatment with medication. Although clinicians often feel frustrated by the seriousness of the patient's resistance and denial, threatening or

Table 6–1. Elements of a successful medication strategy for treatment of chronically mentally ill patients

Collaborative relationship
Education
Systematic approach to control of symptoms
Assessment of capacity for informed consent
Fostering of autonomy in capable patients
Judicious use of coercive strategies when necessary
Awareness of the psychotherapeutic meanings of medication use

bullying a patient into taking medication is unlikely to be successful. The clinician may have to work with the patient and family through several relapses and hospitalizations before the patient can accept the necessity for continued medication, as in the following example:

> Susan Stern was a 19-year-old college freshman when she suffered her first psychotic episode. A tall, attractive, intellectually gifted woman, she has had great difficulty accepting the reality of her psychotic illness. Her accomplished and ambitious parents join her in minimizing its severity.
>
> She responded well to moderate doses of neuroleptic medication. After discharge from the hospital she was followed in outpatient treatment, and after 4 months she resumed her college studies. After 6 months both Susan and her parents began to express concern about the risk of TD and its potentially disfiguring effects, and to insist on tapering her medication. Over the subsequent 2 months she gradually became more irritable, preoccupied, and withdrawn, and complained of sleep disturbance and of difficulty concentrating. When her clinician suggested that these complaints might be prodromal psychotic symptoms, she insisted that they were normal and understandable responses to the stress of returning to college. One month later she was rehospitalized with recurrent psychotic symptoms.
>
> During the second hospitalization Ms. Stern and her parents were able to acknowledge that medication had been discontinued prematurely. They agreed that long-term treatment with medication would be necessary, and Ms. Stern was discharged on a modest maintenance neuroleptic dose. However, a year later, the parents again began to question whether their daughter might be able to do well on a reduced dose of medication. At their insistence, the dosage of medication was gradually reduced, but after 2 months Ms. Stern again began to have prodromal psychotic symptoms. This time she was able to recognize the symptoms herself, and she asked that the doses of medication be increased. Although she had a period of increased symptoms and shaky function, hospitalization was not necessary this time, and Ms. Stern has been conscientious since then about taking her prescribed medication.

In this example, the physician's patient collaboration with Susan and her parents allows them to persuade themselves of the necessity for continued medication compliance. Unfortunately, this strategy is effective only in patients who are sufficiently accepting of their illness and well enough organized at baseline to be able to learn from the experience of relapse.

For patients who are more disorganized, collaboration may focus on the acceptance of depot medication as a joint strategy for facilitating compliance. Depot medication can also encourage collaboration by eliminating uncertainty about how much medication the patient is actually taking.

Arthur Trumbull, a 29-year-old man with schizophrenia, begins to skip doses of oral medication and is becoming psychotic. His psychiatrist, whom he has been seeing for 2 years, recommends a switch to depot medication as a means of strengthening the therapeutic alliance:

> DOCTOR: The work we have been doing together cannot proceed unless both of us can be certain you are taking enough medication. You are counting on my help with dealing with your family and returning to work, but I can't help you if I'm not sure of your medication dosage; otherwise I can't be certain you won't get sick again.

The patient, persuaded that the psychiatrist really cared about him, accepted the medication change.

Even patients in denial can sometimes be engaged in a collaborative relationship to promote medication compliance. Such collaboration, as in the following example, requires the physician to be flexible enough to support the patient's agenda as well as his or her own:

Ms. Grimes, a 60-year-old woman with paranoid schizophrenia, continues to deny that she has a mental illness. She views her main problems as an inability to find an affordable apartment and a lack of support from her children. Her psychiatrist, who had originally committed her and initiated involuntary medication because she could not care for herself, has persuaded her that voluntary compliance with depot medication would facilitate her discharge. Following discharge to a rooming house, the patient agrees to continue medication compliance in return for her physician's help in finding her an affordable apartment and in serving as a liaison to her children. She also knows that lack of compliance and cooperation may result in another commitment.

Education

The task of educating patients and family members begins as early as possible in the patient's course of treatment. Concerns about the disturbing side effects of high doses of antipsychotic medications should be acknowledged; the patient and family should be reassured that the medication dose will be reduced as soon as the clinical situation permits and that the "preventive dose" of the medication will be designed to minimize side effects.

Education of patients and families can focus on anticipated areas of resistance, both early in treatment and later, as the same questions keep arising. Some typical questions—and possible answers—are listed below:

PATIENT 1: How long must I take medicine? Forever?

RESIDENT: You may not have to take antipsychotic medication forever. Many patients do get to the point where they no longer need medicine or require very low doses, but it can take a long time. The best strategy for now is to continue to take medication as prescribed, at least for the next year, to prevent a relapse that could set you back. We can evaluate your need to continue medicine on a year-to-year basis.

* * *

PATIENT 2: What is tardive dyskinesia, and what are the chances I will get it?

RESIDENT: Tardive dyskinesia is a possible long-term effect of medication that occurs in a few patients, generally only after many years of being on medication. The usual symptoms are involuntary mouth, tongue, finger, hand, and leg movements that can range from being mild and barely noticeable to being, in rare cases, severe and disabling. Rarely—in fewer than 1 out of 1,000 cases—severe body spasms can also occur. In most patients, early detection and reduction of medication will get rid of the symptoms. In a small number of patients, however, the symptoms do not go away.

It is most important, however, to weigh the relatively small risk of TD against the nearly certain likelihood of relapse without medication. You need to be fully informed about both the dangers of taking medicine and the dangers of not taking medicine so that you can understand why we want you to continue to take it.

* * *

PATIENT 3: What will happen if I stop the medicine? How can you be sure I will relapse?

RESIDENT: If you have had only one episode of psychosis and you have completely cleared up, it is worth a try—after about a year—to stop medicine gradually and see what happens. When you first stop medicine, you are likely to feel better, because the side effects go away before the antipsychotic effects do. This does not mean you do not need medication! The risk of relapse is often highest 3 to 6 months after a reduction in medication, so continued monitoring after the medicine is stopped is very important. We must wait and see if you will relapse, and be prepared to start the medicine again immediately at the earliest indication of trouble. On the other hand, if you have already had relapses caused by discontinuing or reducing medicine, it is just about certain that you will relapse again. I therefore would insist that you continue medication indefinitely, and not take chances on going backwards by risking relapse.

* * *

PATIENT 4: If the medicine still makes me feel terrible, why should I take it?

RESIDENT: Antipsychotic medicines have many uncomfortable side effects that, unfortunately, cannot always be completely eliminated by side-effect medication. The best strategy for reducing side effects is maintaining strict medication compliance and working with me on different trials of side-effect medications and on careful adjustment of medication dosages. A comfortable medication regimen can almost always be achieved with patience. However, if some side effects ultimately cannot be eliminated, we must work together on helping you to accept them as the best possible result for now, and not frustrate yourself by trying to feel "perfect" when you have a very serious illness.

By the same token, much of the discomfort you feel when you are on medications is due to the illness, not due to the meds. Slow thinking, persistent confusion, difficulty working, paranoia, voices, and so on are due to the illness. Without meds, these symptoms would be worse, not better, once the meds wear off. This is painful for most people to face, and it may help you to talk with me from time to time about how it feels to be persistently symptomatic and disabled, even when on medicine. I wish the meds could do a better job, but they can't, and you and I need to deal with that together.

Systematic Approach to the Control of Symptoms

For symptoms and side effects that are refractory to the initial medication regimen, it helps the resident to have a patient, systematic approach to achieving maximum symptom relief. Elements of such a systematic approach are outlined in Table 6–2.

For schizophrenia, as of 1992, a trial of three antipsychotics from different categories (e.g., phenothiazines, thiothixenes, and butyrophenones), along with the systematic addition of lithium, carbamazepine, and clonazepam or lorazepam, is generally considered adequate. When possible, a trial of clozapine must always be considered for refractory patients. Note that a systematic sequence of medication trials may take years, so patience and careful analysis are crucial. Ultimately, in refractory cases, the physician needs to recognize when the disruptive impact of continued medication changes outweighs the benefit of simply sticking with an established, although imperfect, regimen. Often, progress in rehabilitation cannot occur until the patient accepts that his or her disability will not be fixed by further medicine "magic," and begins the painful work of facing the limitations imposed by the chronic mental illness.

Assessment of Capacity for Informed Consent

In order to participate collaboratively with patients and families in a medication treatment relationship, the clinician must obtain informed consent

Table 6–2. Elements of a systematic approach to control of symptoms in chronically mentally ill patients

1. Increase first line drug(s) until maximum beneficial effect is obtained.
2. Measure levels, if possible, to ensure therapeutic dose and compliance.
3. If compliance is in doubt, use depot medication(s) and/or frequent levels.
4. Take enough time to ensure maximum therapeutic benefit and adequate assessment of effect (usually, 1 to 3 months, although bipolar disorder may require a full-year cycle).
5. Follow the same sequential steps for each additional first-line, second-line, or third-line drug tried.
6. Change only one drug at a time whenever possible.
7. Follow the same steps for each illness or target symptom.
8. Do not try to eliminate all discomfort, anxiety, or depression.
9. Be patient.

from the patient and/or family members. This requirement complicates an already formidable education task. Although obtaining informed consent is essential, the clinician should take the patient's mental state into consideration in determining when and how to discuss medication's risks and benefits. If the clinician concludes that the patient is too acutely disturbed to make a competent judgment about the matter, he or she may decide to defer obtaining full informed consent until the patient is better able to understand the available choices. In such instances informed consent should be obtained from a family member, who should also be informed of the reasons for delaying obtaining consent from the patient.

In some instances, however, the patient's persistent psychotic symptoms and/or denial of illness may preclude his or her ever being able to provide informed consent or to provide it consistently. In other patients, understanding and insight about their need for medication fluctuate from week to week, day to day, or even hour to hour.

Matthew Jermyn (continued from p. 83)

When Mr. Jermyn is discharged from the hospital, he appears to understand his illness and the need for ongoing medication, and to appreciate his parents' willingness to set limits to ensure his compliance. A few months later, however, he abruptly refuses medicine. When Dr. Transome assesses Mr. Jermyn's competence to make an informed refusal, Mr. Jermyn replies that he no longer needs medicine because he is no longer ill, and in fact had never been ill; his "illness" is all a plot cooked up by his parents and the doctor. This delusional construct satisfies Dr. Transome that Mr. Jermyn is not competent to make an informed decision at this time. Dr. Transome knows that Mr. Jermyn's bouts of paranoia usually do not last long, but he also knows that if the paranoia leads Mr. Jermyn to stop medication, Mr. Jermyn will decompensate. Dr. Transome believes that it is essential to keep the patient on medicine through the periods of "temporary incompetence" to prevent further deterioration.

In other patients, the inability to provide informed consent can be a chronic problem, as is seen in the following case:

Mr. Thorpe

Mr. Thorpe was committed to the hospital with a first episode of paranoid schizophrenia, during which he threatened neighbors with a knife for beaming "emasculation rays" at him. During his hospitalization, he steadfastly denied illness, taking medication only when a temporary guardianship was obtained through a court order. Even after his psychosis cleared to the point where he could be discharged, Mr. Thorpe's psychotic denial continued so that he refused medication and the paranoid symptoms returned. Despite massive efforts by his family, his psychiatrist, and the hospital staff to educate him about his illness, his denial persisted even after three episodes of relapse and recompensation.

In such instances, obtaining informed consent is simply impossible.

As these examples indicate, the resident needs first to assess each case to ascertain the extent to which the patient is capable, temporarily incapable, or chronically incapable of providing informed consent. If the patient is capable of consent and collaboration, the resident should try to foster as much autonomy as possible; if the patient is temporarily or intermittently incapable of consent, then depot administration, family supervision and/or contracting, or staff supervision should be instituted. If, however, the patient is chronically incapable of informed consent, legal enforcement of compliance may be necessary.

Fostering Autonomy

Although in the short term, psychotic patients may benefit from being cajoled, coerced, or even forced to take medication, the ultimate goal for chronically ill patients is to encourage as much autonomy as possible. In the long term, maximizing autonomy allows the patient to internalize the need for medication and thus to collaborate with the physician in the medication process. Patients whose compliance depends solely on external pressure are likely to stop medication as soon as the external pressure relents.

The difficulty for the resident is deciding how far to let a patient go who is making decisions with which the resident does not agree. The resident's assessment of the patient's capacity to provide informed consent will be an important determinant of this decision.

Use of Coercive Strategies

For patients who are unwilling or unable to maintain medication compliance, the resident will have to use coercive strategies. As with Dr. Transome in the opening vignette of this chapter, this process can arouse conflict in the resident, who experiences the ethical dilemma of choosing between feeling guilty about invading the patient's rights and watching helplessly as the patient decompensates. Many residents find that they cannot bring themselves to use coercion of any type until they have seen for themselves the deleterious effects of repeated noncompliance and relapse in patients who do not seem to learn from these experiences. Because many such patients get worse after each episode of relapse, more aggressive medication strategies are usually indicated.

An elaborate and otherwise apparently well-designed plan can fail if any one of the following elements is missing.

Enforcement. Mr. Jermyn's parents made his compliance with im fluphenazine a condition of returning home and remaining at home. When he refused his shot, however, the Jermyns were unwilling to insist that he leave.

Another patient, under medication guardianship, was also receiving im fluphenazine. When he refused his shot, no plan was in place to administer medication involuntarily.

Assessment of compliance. A patient orally taking trifluoperazine and lithium carbonate was required to be medication compliant to remain at his parents' home. When he began to decompensate his parents suspected noncompliance. The patient insisted that he was compliant and brought in empty medication containers as "proof." The patient later admitted that he was dumping his medicine down the sink.

Circumvention of psychiatrist participation. Because of noncompliance on orally administered medications, a patient at a community residence was required to take im haloperidol as prescribed by her mental health center psychiatrist as a condition for remaining in the residence. However, after consultation with a private psychiatrist, who prescribed oral medication, the patient "fired" the mental health center psychiatrist, became noncompliant, and relapsed.

Caregiver cooperation. Parents of a schizophrenic young woman insisted that she comply with im medication for her to remain at home. The patient's sister, who lived nearby, thought that the parents were unfair, so whenever they attempted to enforce the contract, the sister took the patient in.

The following are some examples of successful coercive strategies. The first example describes a contract to take im medication as a contingency of failed compliance with oral medicine:

> Virginia Clark, a 42-year-old married woman with schizophrenia, is hospitalized after decompensation due to noncompliance with oral perphenazine. Intramuscular fluphenazine is proposed, but the patient refuses, saying that she has "learned her lesson." She also acknowledges that the akathisia side effects of fluphenazine had made her very uncomfortable in the past. Her husband supports her and wants her to have "one more chance." The psychiatrist proposes a contract requiring that if she relapses again due to medication noncompliance, both the psychiatrist and the husband will insist on im medication(s).
>
> The patient signs the contract, but after doing well for 9 months, she gradually and surreptitiously discontinues her perphenazine so that she ultimately relapses. After she is hospitalized and restabilized, she reluctantly agrees to take im fluphenazine, but only in small doses. She has now been maintained successfully for a year on fluphenazine decanoate, 2.5 mg (0.1 cc) im every 2–3 weeks.

In the next example, the patient does not comply until faced with enforcement of the contingencies:

> Josephine Barker is a 41-year-old woman with a long history of paranoid schizophrenia who has required over 20 state hospitalizations. After recompensating she would always return home to her parents, who never had agreed to enforce medication compliance.
>
> During one of the patient's hospitalizations, the parents were persuaded by a son to stop accepting Ms. Barker back into their home. So when the patient's condition clears, the parents for the first time refuse to take her home.
>
> The psychiatrist asks them if they would take the patient home under the condition she would take im medication. The parents agree,

but when this plan is presented to the patient, she screams: "You can't let them do this. That stuff will kill me. You gotta take me home." When the parents say nothing, the psychiatrist tells the patient that as she does not agree with the plan, the meeting is over, and she will remain in the hospital until another meeting can be scheduled. The patient looks around for a moment, then sits down calmly and says, "O.K., I'll take the shots. Now, what else do I have to do?"

Now, 2 years later, the patient remains out of the state hospital and continues to take im fluphenazine.

In another example, compliance with orally administered medicine is a requirement for referral to rehabilitative services:

Helen Metcalf, a 35-year-old woman with bipolar disorder, is erratic with lithium compliance. She attends therapy regularly, hoping to address her mood swings in psychotherapy. She cannot hold a job, but when she demands referral to a supported employment program, she is told that, because of her history, she will first have to demonstrate 6 months of lithium compliance, documented by periodic blood levels. The patient readily agrees, later acknowledging that she knew she needed to stay on lithium, but that she needed someone to tell her she had to.

In a final example, persistent efforts to obtain a medication guardianship eventually pay off:

Mr. Thorpe (continued from p. 93)

Mr. Thorpe has maintained his denial of his illness despite three relapses. However, his family—parents and siblings—have gradually become convinced that the psychiatrist is right and that medication compliance is necessary, so the father agrees to apply to the court for a medication guardianship.

At first, the judge grants only a 90-day order, advising the patient to follow through voluntarily after the order expires. However, when the patient again refuses medicine, relapses, and returns to the same judge, the judge grants a permanent order. When Mr. Thorpe still refuses to comply, he is told that if he does not take the medicine voluntarily, he could be committed to the hospital until he agrees to take his shot. Mr. Thorpe tests this procedure twice before accepting medication.

Once he is taking medicine regularly, under guardianship, Mr. Thorpe begins to work with the psychiatrist. During the next year, his biweekly fluphenazine is gradually reduced, he has fewer side effects, and he is able to get a full-time job. He tells the psychiatrist: "I don't agree with you that I am schizophrenic. But I can see why you thought so because of all those crazy ideas I had."

Assessment of Meanings of Medication Use

Medication is so important in treatment that it usually acquires a variety of personal meanings. For example, a patient may casually remark, as he leaves at the end of a psychotherapeutic session, "By the way, I'm not sure, but I might need a renewal of my prescription." The clinician not only should make certain that the patient has enough medication, but also should note and, if possible, explore the underlying meaning of the incident. In this instance, the patient appears to be testing the clinician's view of the necessity of medication compliance, perhaps as a manifestation of the patient's wish to deny his illness and to shift responsibility for his treatment onto the psychiatrist.

For many patients, taking medication challenges their autonomy and leads them to feel controlled rather than cared for. In the following vignette, the patient's anger at the resident's vacation takes the form of refusal of medication:

> PATIENT: I'm really bothered by my voices, and all you ever do is give me Prolixin. I'm sick and tired of being controlled by your medicines. While I'm suffering, you're enjoying yourself on vacation. You probably get a fat kickback from the drug company. This Prolixin does me no good at all. If you cared at all about how I feel, you'd stop it! I'm not going to take my shot any more.
>
> RESIDENT: I understand that you feel deserted when I'm on vacation, and that you feel angry that you're suffering while I'm having a good time. But I do care about you, and, in fact, I would be irresponsible and uncaring if I stopped your medicine. Remember the last time we tried to lower your dosage and you got much worse? I know you hate it that the medicine doesn't eliminate the voices, but you'd be much worse without it.
>
> PATIENT: Well, maybe. I suppose you could look at it like that. O.K., I suppose I'll take it—for now.

Other patients, believing that giving medicine is the only way for the resident to show concern for them, insist on medicine for anxiety, depression, headaches, and so on. The resident needs to assess to what extent these symptoms require medication and to what extent they require psychological intervention. Most chronic patients have good reason to experience depression and anxiety, and they need to learn nonpharmacological methods for processing these experiences. In general, once a patient has been stabilized on a maintenance dose of medication, changes should be infrequent and part of an overall strategy of medication management.

Decisions about prescribing medication may also reflect the resident's impatience or discomfort with the patient, which may lead the resident to prescribe more medicine or a new medicine rather than to sit with the patient and listen to his or her painful feelings. Conversely, anger at a patient's denial may lead the resident to accede to discontinuing medication rather than to develop a strategy for ensuring compliance.

Matthew Jermyn (continued from p. 93)

Dr. Transome realizes that Mr. Jermyn's psychotic denial is interfering with both his compliance and his competence. He also suspects that, down deep, Mr. Jermyn is testing whether his parents and Dr. Transome really care enough to face the painful reality of his illness with him by enforcing the treatment contract. Dr. Transome decides to set up a meeting with the patient's parents.

In the meeting, Dr. Transome listens carefully to the Jermyns. They are afraid to confront their son, reluctant to evict him, and still wish that perhaps the medication is not really necessary. Dr. Transome patiently addresses each issue in turn. He reviews Mr. Jermyn's 10 previous decompensations, each precipitated by medication refusal, and observes that he has been getting worse after each decompensation. He explains that Mr. Jermyn, like many other patients, appears to be testing to see if all of them—parents and doctor—care enough to follow through. Finally, Dr. Transome makes it clear that they do not have to kick their son out permanently and that he can return home as soon as he gets his shot. Further, Dr. Transome agrees to arrange shelter or hospitalization if necessary.

With Dr. Transome's support, the Jermyns agree to confront Matthew about the necessity to remain medication compliant if he wishes to live at home. When they do so, Matthew becomes highly agitated. "Fine. If that's how you feel, I'll leave!" he screams, and runs out of the office. Dr. Transome offers him a shelter or hospital, but Matthew says, "Don't worry. I know how to survive."

The Jermyns are distraught. Dr. Transome reassures them that their son will probably show up at the emergency room that night, although inwardly he is concerned that he might have "blown it." The police are called to look for Mr. Jermyn, but he is nowhere to be found.

The next morning, Mr. Jermyn shows up at the emergency room. "I want my shot so I can go home!" he announces. He reports that he spent the night in the woods. Even though he looks as if he had had a horrible night, he says, "It was fine in the woods; I can handle it, but I think I'd rather live at home."

Mr. Jermyn then receives his shot, returns home, and stops testing the limits on his medication compliance.

7

Individual Psychotherapy With Chronically Mentally Ill Patients

Although not all chronically mentally ill patients benefit from individual psychotherapy, the treatment plans for the four patients discussed in Chapter 5 included a component of individual psychotherapy. For Mr. Maddox, Mr. Jermyn, and Ms. DeBarry, the psychotherapy was provided by the resident, while other members of the treatment team provided individual treatment for Ms. Hogarth. In all four cases the psychotherapeutic treatment differed, particularly in flexibility, from the traditional psychotherapy provided to nonpsychotic patients.

Chronically psychotic patients vary greatly, at times dramatically and unpredictably, and even a familiar patient will have changing needs and varying presentations as treatment proceeds.

Basic Structure of Treatment

Length and Frequency of Sessions

Flexibility begins with decisions about the length and frequency of sessions. Although some chronically psychotic patients can make excellent use of frequent, regular, hour-long sessions, others may be unable to tolerate the intensity and stimulation of a full hour's contact, no matter how supportive and gentle the therapist is.

Often the best way to determine the most appropriate structure for the treatment is to ask the patient what seems comfortable and to observe his or her tolerance for sessions of various lengths. Mr. Maddox, for example, said that he wished to meet no more than 30 minutes every other week. Mr. Jermyn wished to meet weekly, but could not tolerate sessions longer than 30 minutes, whereas Ms. DeBarry expected a full 50 minutes each week. Ms. Hogarth, the most limited and disorganized of the four, did best with frequent, short sessions, such as 15 minutes twice a week, held in her workshop program rather than in an office.

Some patients, unfortunately, find it hard to state clearly their reactions to psychotherapy. Thus, a patient who finds the psychotherapeutic hours too intense may not say so, but may instead respond by missing sessions, by being late, by coming to the sessions intoxicated, or by complaining incessantly about the therapist, the medication, or the treatment. In such situations, flexibility is particularly important, as in the following example:

> Mr. Rubins, a 23-year-old man with a 4-year history of psychotic illness, regularly comes at least 20 minutes late to his weekly individual psychotherapy hour. When his resident gently points this out to him, Mr. Rubins mentions that though he plans to come on time, something always comes up to delay him. Noting that Mr. Rubins is anxious and uncomfortable during the sessions, the resident suggests that half-hour sessions might be more useful. Mr. Rubins soon begins coming on time for most sessions.

Therapist Behavior

Chronically psychotic patients ordinarily feel stigmatized and socially unappealing, and they are usually exquisitely sensitive to any real or imagined sign of rejection. Especially in the early sessions, therefore, it helps to be friendly as well as professional, active without being intrusive, and alert and responsive to the patient's anxieties and concerns, even when these are irrational. Questions prompted by the patient's anxiety need unequivocal answers rather than interpretations.

Matthew Jermyn (continued from p. 98)

> Entering Dr. Transome's outpatient office for the first time, Mr. Jermyn looks carefully around the room. He stares intently at the intercom on the wall and asks, "Is that your secret tape recorder?" Dr. Transome responds with a question, "What made you think I might be recording our sessions?" This response causes Mr. Jermyn to become so terrified and suspicious that he runs out of the session. Dr. Transome follows after him, reassures him with some difficulty, and helps him to return.

Reflecting on the interchange, Dr. Transome realizes he would have done better to answer Mr. Jermyn's question with a simple "No, that's the intercom, and it's shut off now."

Many psychotic patients are vigilant and sensitive observers, although they frequently misinterpret the significance of their observations. Questions or responses that stem from such hyperalert observations require open and reassuring responses. For example, Ms. DeBarry began a session by saying, "Doctor Lyon, you seem annoyed today." Dr. Lyon responded, "Yes, I am a bit annoyed about something that happened earlier, but it has nothing to do with you." Ms. DeBarry relaxed and was able to let the matter drop. Such a response validates the patient's perception but at the same time corrects a possible misinterpretation.

Being warm and friendly—assuming the therapist is in fact a warm and friendly person—does not mean that the therapist should be effusive or overly chummy. The goal is to help put the patient at ease, not to pretend to be close friends.

Content of Sessions

Psychotherapy with the chronically psychotic patient at first looks deceptively like an ordinary conversation. The clinician is comparatively active, contributing ideas and opinions and expressing emotions in moderation. It is usually wise to keep the focus on current feelings, issues related to acceptance of the illness, and practical problems and concerns. The following case illustrates this point:

Mr. Matthews is a constricted, intellectualizing college student who is surprisingly intact as a young adult even though he had developed schizophrenia as a child. He begins outpatient psychotherapy with an enthusiastic resident who is determined to deal psychotherapeutically with as much as he can. He gives Mr. Matthews the "standard" instructions to tell him everything that comes to mind without censoring.

Mr. Matthews readily complies. Within a few sessions he relates a dream of having sex with his mother. When the resident proceeds to ask for the patient's associations to the dream, he is told of some bloody and violent thoughts. Still thinking Mr. Matthews is a "good" psychotherapy patient, he pursues these bizarre trains of thought and later tells his supervisor that he believes that the material is related to one of Mr. Matthews' primary complaints: that of being unable to get close to women. The supervisor agrees, but points out that with his past history of schizophrenia, Mr. Matthews needs the structure of a reality focus, and that no matter what the content, the resident should direct the discussion in future sessions toward everyday issues and problem solving, and away from the bizarre material that lurks not far beneath the surface.

Other patients may become disorganized not through the emergence of an underlying psychosis, but as a result of the therapist's focusing on issues that deflect attention from the daily priority of maintaining stability, as in the following example:

Ms. DeBarry (continued from p. 81)

Ms. DeBarry continually devotes much energy in each session to recounting emotionally intense impressions of her somewhat scattered daily activities, at first drawing Dr. Lyon into in-depth discussions of the "psychodynamic" meanings of her various associations and ideas. Dr. Lyon quickly learns, however, that pursuing these avenues leads nowhere, but instead represents the patient's resistances to focusing on the more mundane and depressing reality of managing her chronic affective disorder, and beginning to examine, and perhaps change, her somewhat empty life. Dr. Lyon finds that simply listening quietly and attentively until Ms. DeBarry finishes her stories, and then redirecting the focus, as by asking her how she is managing with her medicine, is effective in helping Ms. DeBarry to maintain stability.

Much of the work of individual psychotherapy is taken up with gentle, repetitive attempts to educate the patient about the nature of chronic mental illness, and with painstaking negotiations about compliance with the details of treatment. As was the case with Mr. Maddox in the previous chapter, this work is often difficult and slow, and patients are usually resistant:

Ms. Alcott is a 54-year-old woman with a 30-year history of chronic schizophrenia. At her best she is cognitively disorganized, socially isolated, and only marginally able to care for her daily needs. Often, however, her thought disorder will become worse, and she is plagued by threatening auditory hallucinations, paranoid delusions, and referential thoughts. At such times she will stop eating and engage in public displays of bizarre behavior that result in her hospitalization. She has always been treated with orally administered antipsychotic drugs, and her relapses usually follow her forgetting to take her medication because of her chronic cognitive disorganization. During the last 5 years of her illness, her longest period out of the hospital has been 9 months.

After her most recent relapse Ms. Alcott is assigned to Dr. Flannery, a resident at her mental health center. When he recommends a change to a depot form of antipsychotic medication, she refuses, saying that "she doesn't like shots." Dr. Flannery responds by increasing the

> frequency of her appointments and requiring her to bring her pill bottles for pill counts, which diminishes but does not completely resolve the problem. Meanwhile, at each visit Dr. Flannery suggests depot medication and explores and discusses the reasons for her objections. Eventually, after the sixth visit, Ms. Alcott agrees. As a result, she has not needed hospitalization for 2 years.

Residents who enjoy the intricate probing of layers of unconscious processes in psychotherapy may initially view psychotherapy with chronically mentally ill patients as mundane because the content of sessions is so focused on external reality. Actually, however, psychotherapy with chronic patients is not at all mundane: it is often far more intricate, challenging, and subtle than ordinary psychodynamic therapy. In every session, the therapist needs to be tuned in simultaneously to biological issues (i.e., issues of stability of the illness) and to family issues and system issues (i.e., issues regarding the patient's interactions with significant caregivers). At the same time the therapist remains concerned with the patient's individual psychodynamics and individual program of rehabilitation and recovery, continually having to decide whether to discuss these issues openly or leave them alone while keeping up a relaxed, casual conversation focused on day-to-day problems. Such work is neither simple nor straightforward, but it can be the key to whether the patient is to function at all well in the world.

The resident has to be continuously alert to the possibility that the patient may suffer a psychotic decompensation, even when therapy may appear to be proceeding smoothly; if the therapist has reason to suspect that the patient is decompensating, active intervention is required. A telephone call to a patient who has missed a session may help determine if the absence was a manifestation of resistance to treatment or the product of a prodromal psychotic syndrome. In some instances, contact with family members may also help to clarify the situation, and a family meeting may be useful to help mobilize available resources to try to control a developing psychotic decompensation.

Educational efforts are important in order to help the patient understand his or her reactions and feelings about the illness, to monitor his or her inner state, to identify prodromal signs of recurrent illness, and to encourage the patient to take appropriate steps to intervene before an exacerbation of symptoms becomes disabling:

> Ms. Manchester is a 23-year-old woman with a 4-year history of schizoaffective illness. After her first psychotic episode, which occurred midway through her freshman year of college, she worked for a year before returning to school. She was maintained on lithium and a neuroleptic and was fully compliant with treatment. When she re-

turned to college and appeared to be in remission, medication was gradually tapered.

By midsemester break, however, she had developed prodromal symptoms of recurrent psychosis, including sleep disturbance, marked irritability, and paranoid ideation. When her therapist attempted to alert her to these symptoms and to persuade her to take larger doses of medication, she refused, insisting that she was not suffering a relapse. After several weeks, she had to be hospitalized again.

In the hospital, she acknowledged the risk of recurrent psychosis and admitted that she had ignored the warning symptoms. Subsequently, she cooperated more fully in monitoring her psychological state and informing her therapist if she needed an increase in medication.

Another important goal of individual treatment is to suggest and implement strategies for the patient to improve his or her capacity to control or suppress symptoms in order to function in society. In general, the clinician works on this goal in a matter-of-fact, practical way, while maintaining a capacity for creative experimentation, as in the following example:

Mr. Quinn

Mr. Quinn, a 29-year-old man with long-standing schizophrenia, has chronic auditory hallucinations that have not been responsive to fairly high doses of intramuscular fluphenazine. The voices keep telling the patient that he is lazy and a failure, a view with which the patient's mother, a forceful and ambitious woman, agrees. Family psychotherapeutic work has been directed at convincing the mother that putting more pressure on Mr. Quinn is counterproductive, and that he would do better if she backed off. Individual psychotherapy has been directed at helping Mr. Quinn to accept his voices and his disability:

THERAPIST: Are the voices bothering you?

MR. QUINN: Yeah. They're giving me a hard time today.

THERAPIST: How are you coping?

MR. Q.: I keep telling them to be quiet.

THERAPIST: Does it work?

MR. Q.: No. They get louder. They keep telling me I'm a failure.

THERAPIST: And when you try to control them and you can't, you feel like more of a failure—and the voices get louder.

MR. Q.: So what should I do?

THERAPIST: Stop trying to control the voices. The voices are part of your illness. The more you accept your illness, the more comfortable you will feel. When you hear the voices, don't fight; just relax and go on about your business. The voices are a signal that you are under stress, so you may need to slow down.

MR. Q.: But I have to fight. The voices say I'm a failure if I give up.

THERAPIST: The voices get louder when you feel like a failure. Let's see if we can talk about those feelings.

The more Mr. Quinn "surrenders" to the voices and accepts his powerlessness over them, the less they bother him. He is eventually able to be more assertive with his mother, and as a result he can be more helpful at home. After a while he begins to report that he hears "God's voice" telling him to accept himself, take his medication, "take it slow," and do what he can. He finds the new voice very comforting.

Some patients are able to make use of a more exploratory approach:

Ms. Raleigh, a 20-year-old woman with schizophrenia, has heard accusatory voices since age 15. One of the precipitants of her first psychotic episode was her disclosure of sexual abuse by her father. Her parents attacked her for her accusations and consistently denied them, after which she developed auditory hallucinations that told her that she was bad and deserved to die. Her parents reluctantly agreed to her hospitalization, but denied her mental illness; her mother, who had a history of paranoid psychosis, kept telling Ms. Raleigh that she was making up the voices and that she was a drug addict for taking medicine.

Inevitably, Ms. Raleigh discontinued her medications and gradually deteriorated until she needed rehospitalization. Now that she is back on medication, she slowly begins to improve, until her mother visits and once again attacks her for taking drugs. The next day Ms. Raleigh's voices are again worse, telling her she is "bad." In psychotherapy, her psychiatrist focuses on trying to help her to understand what has happened:

THERAPIST: How are the voices today?

MS. RALEIGH: Very bad. They say I'm bad.

THERAPIST: Do you have any idea what made them worse?

MS. R. [*passively*]: No.

THERAPIST: Think for a minute.

[*Ms. Raleigh shrugs helplessly.*]

THERAPIST: Well, what makes your voices worse in general?

MS. R.: I don't know.

THERAPIST: Sure you do. Give yourself a minute and it will come to you.

MS. R. [*pausing first*]: . . . Maybe stress?

THERAPIST: Yes. Like what, for example?

MS. R.: My family. Thinking about the past. Also if I smoke pot.

THERAPIST: Do any of these apply in the last day or so?

MS. R.: Well, I saw my mother yesterday.

THERAPIST: How did it go?

MS. R.: Not good. She told me to stop my meds—that I was faking it and wasn't really sick.

THERAPIST: How did that make you feel?

MS. R.: Bad.

THERAPIST: Guilty?

MS. R.: Yes.

THERAPIST: So the voices got louder and told you you're a bad person?

MS. R.: Yes.

Ms. Raleigh demonstrates how the symptoms of a basically biological illness, schizophrenia, can be precipitated and its course affected by psychosocial stress. Without the biological predisposition, Ms. Raleigh may well have responded to the stresses in her life with an emotional illness, but it would not have been schizophrenia.

The following is another example of a careful, gentle exploratory approach, focusing on current problems and concerns:

Sally Weston, a 46-year-old married woman, has had numerous hospitalizations for psychotic episodes over the past 15 years. She has been out of the hospital for 30 months, and, although on fairly high doses of psychoactive medications, she continues to have ideas of reference and, at times, paranoid delusions. When especially upset, she is certain that everyone is saying she is a lesbian.

Many of her early weekly sessions with the therapist center on helping her identify the ideas of reference and delusions as symptoms—indicators that she is anxious and under pressure. She is at first skeptical, but because she has a positive relationship with her therapist, she is willing to entertain the idea. After four or five sessions, she is able to say, "I must tell you that I understand all this on an intellectual level, but I'm not sure I really believe it down deep. Since I trust you, I'll operate as if I really believed it." By examining her symptoms each time they occur, she is able, with the therapist's help, to identify the particular stress that has precipitated them and to formulate a course of action that will resolve the situation. By dealing with her symptoms in this way, she finds that her life is becoming less chaotic and more enjoyable, and her condition does not deteriorate to the point where her symptoms become fixed paranoid delusions.

After 6 months of this kind of work in therapy, she is able to talk about her delusion that people were saying that she was a lesbian, and to recognize that at such times her anxiety was especially severe. She is relieved by understanding that the symptoms indicated anxiety rather than real and incomprehensible threats that were utterly beyond her control.

Working Toward Rehabilitation

An important component of long-term individual therapy with chronically mentally ill patients is helping them to work on the "next step" in the process of rehabilitation. In this stage, patients are helped to overcome the negative symptoms of passivity and lack of motivation that are often related to feelings of helplessness, inadequacy, and despair. Patients are also helped to relinquish grandiose and unattainable goals, which often reflect narcissistic defenses against recognizing the severity of their disability, and to accept the necessity of the slow pace of progress by setting realistic and attainable objectives. Part of this process involves knowing how and when to refer the patient to community resources and rehabilitation programs. (This aspect will be discussed more fully in Chapter 9.)

Mr. Parker

Mr. Parker, a 28-year-old man with schizophrenia, has begun treatment in the outpatient clinic at the urging of his parents, who are fed up with his immobility and lack of progress. In the initial sessions, Mr. Parker, who is adequately stabilized on trifluoperazine and lithium, reveals that he enjoys spending his time lying in his room fantasizing about a woman whom he had met 5 years earlier in a bar. Although he had had no further contact with her, he had elaborated a delusional fantasy that she was seriously interested in him and was waiting until he "got on his feet" so that she could marry him.

With regard to "getting on his feet," Mr. Parker says that he can't work currently because he doesn't feel like himself "yet," but that when he does have a good day, he can "lick the world." He is waiting more or less patiently for the good days to start happening consistently. He tells the therapist of a lucrative family business, which was begun by his grandfather, that has now passed to his father, and because he is his grandfather's namesake, he is waiting for the business to be handed over to him. In the meantime, he is collecting disability and living in his parents' home.

Although the resident is tempted to berate Mr. Parker for his passivity and to urge him to "get moving" and "face reality," she realizes that this would be a mistake. Instead, she conveys to Mr. Parker that she respects and empathizes with his views and choices, while gently exploring his decision not to pursue more attainable goals. She discovers that his grandiosity, fantasies, and passivity protect him from enormous feelings of inadequacy and failure. She lets him know that she understands how he feels, but that she herself feels more hopeful and positive about his abilities than he does. She suggests that he has nothing to lose by trying a new approach, provided he could trust her to guide him in a way that would protect him from failure.

Gradually, over a period of 6 months, Mr. Parker gives up his fantasied girlfriend and agrees to participate in a simple behavior contract to perform routine chores at home in return for pay. When he is successful in this plan, he begins to believe that he might be able to manage a supported work placement.

Immobilized patients frequently experience enormous pressure from their families to get moving. The therapist, who may empathize with the family's frustration, at the same time needs to convey to the patient and to the family the importance of maintaining the patient's slow pace of progress.

Thomas Maddox (continued from p. 77)

Mr. Maddox's father is impatient with his son's lack of progress in day treatment. Mr. Maddox expresses in therapy both anger at his father's lack of understanding and impatience with himself for not doing more. Dr. Wilcox patiently and repeatedly reminds Mr. Maddox that he is doing the best he can for now, and that simply maintaining a behavior contract at home and attending day treatment is, for him, a monumental achievement. Dr. Wilcox also points out that it is hard for Mr. Maddox to give himself enough credit for how hard he is working, because he has to contend every day with schizophrenia. When Mr. Maddox realizes that his self-imposed pressure is aggravating his psychotic symptoms, he can justify to himself that he has to slow down. In subsequent sessions, he ventilates appropriately to Dr. Wilcox his strong feelings of anger and sadness that he cannot get better any faster.

The process of therapy in the rehabilitative phase requires much sensitivity to the fragility of the patient's self-esteem. The therapist needs to help the patient mourn his or her inability to attain "normal" goals for education, employment, marriage, and family, while at the same time convey consistent hope that if the patient follows a slow, step-by-step process of rehabilitation, considerable progress can be achieved.

A major concern of therapy is helping patients to continue to follow a program of maintaining medication compliance as they progress in rehabilitation. Many patients' anxieties about moving forward take the form of increased denial, flight into health, and discontinuation or reduction of medication, as in the case of Ms. DeBarry:

Ms. DeBarry (continued from p. 102)

After approximately 1 year of consistent therapy with Dr. Lyon, Ms. DeBarry starts to attend a supported work program. Soon thereafter she begins to complain about medications, side effects, and Dr. Lyon's competence as a physician, complaints that Dr. Lyon has not heard for months. Dr. Lyon finds that Ms. DeBarry's lithium level and valproate level are low. "How can I work with all that junk you prescribe messing up my system?" demands Ms. DeBarry. Dr. Lyon stifles his impulse to lecture Ms. DeBarry on medication compliance, saying, "You're worried that you won't do well in the program if you stick with your meds." Ms. DeBarry agrees and calms somewhat. Dr. Lyon then can explore Ms. DeBarry's anxieties about failing, not just because of medication but because of her illness and her feelings of inadequacy. After a while, Ms. DeBarry is able to say, "I guess by not taking my meds I'm setting myself up to fail. That way, if I don't do well I can blame you or the meds—anything but myself."

In other instances, the patient may use treatment noncompliance as a signal that too much is being expected and that any proposed changes should be postponed:

Mary Hogarth (continued from p. 82)

After several months of successfully working a part-time schedule in her sheltered workshop, Ms. Hogarth is asked by her counselor how she would feel about increasing her hours. Ms. Hogarth announces that this is a wonderful idea, saying that she needs to save up money for a trip to Mexico. Ms. Hogarth's counselor suggests that perhaps they should think it over and discuss it again in a few days.

The next day, Ms. Hogarth announces that she has discarded all her pills. Her counselor apologizes for suggesting Ms. Hogarth could handle an increased schedule, and Ms. Hogarth agrees, with inner relief but with outward reluctance, to resume her medication.

Emotional Reactions During Treatment

Dependent Transference

Chronically psychotic patients are able to form intense attachments to their clinicians, although they often have difficulty recognizing or acknowledging the importance of the relationship. Clinicians can also underestimate the importance of the relationship, especially when the patient is emotionally constricted and inexpressive. The clinician should not assume that the patient is indifferent and unattached just because he or she appears to be that way. Apparent indifference usually covers great sensitivity to anticipated rejection, which means that the patient should be informed well in advance about any changes in schedule or absences of the therapist.

Changes in the therapist's attitudes or level of interest may have striking effects on the patient's stability and mood. As the therapy deepens and intensifies, the transference may become especially intense, and the patient may develop a psychotic attachment, as in the following case:

> Ms. Simmons, a 22-year-old chronically schizophrenic patient, appears, suitcase in hand, on her therapist's doorstep on the eve of his vacation. She announces, "I'm moving in. We're getting married!" The therapist, quite appropriately, treats this episode as an expression of the patient's distress and jealousy about his impending vacation with his family.

Many chronic patients are intensely interested in the private lives of their therapists. They may frequently drive by the therapist's house for a look, and even peek through the windows, and they may make "crisis" phone calls at deliberately inconvenient times. The therapist may feel invaded and threatened by interest of this intensity and should address the issue with the patient directly but calmly to establish appropriate distance and boundaries. The patient is more likely to accept the boundary if it is established without superimposing a painful sense of guilt and rejection.

> Ms. Leeds, a 27-year-old woman with chronic schizophrenia, lives independently, supports herself, and makes excellent use of intensive individual treatment. As time goes on, however, she becomes progressively more attached to her therapist and increasingly curious about his private life. She begins walking the streets of his neighborhood each evening to look in the windows of his house and watch him with his family.
>
> After several weeks, Ms. Leeds calls her therapist late one evening to report that she is stranded near his home and that she has no money and no way of getting home. Although she clearly wants her therapist, after having picked her up, to take her home, he takes her to a bus stop and loans her the bus fare.
>
> During the next session, Ms. Leeds is able to describe her fantasy of becoming a silent part of her therapist's family. The therapist responds by asking her to stop her secret spying on his family, saying that they are uncomfortable with her disturbing their privacy. Ms. Leeds asks if she can walk by the house on occasion if she asks permission first, and the therapist agrees.

In general, as treatment progresses, the clinician should expect that the patient will become increasingly attached and dependent. As long as this attachment is a constructive force, motivating the patient to work hard in the therapy, it is a valuable and useful aspect of the therapeutic relationship. It differs from nonpsychotic therapeutic transference both because of its intensity and because psychotic patients can easily lose track of the usual boundaries of the professional relationship. Boundary problems are best handled by explicit, nonjudgmental discussion of each issue as it arises, with the clinician's expectations about appropriate boundaries made clear to the patient at each point.

When the intensity of psychotic transference makes individual treatment unworkable, the patient is better treated in a group or milieu setting, where the transference is diluted among a number of people. The following case illustrates this approach:

> Frances Calloway, a 49-year-old single paranoid schizophrenic woman, has had many hospitalizations since age 22. She has received outpatient treatment over the years at various clinics and has complied with neuroleptic medications. At age 43 she began seeing a private psychiatrist for an hour a week in his office and continued her medications. Within 6 months she became extremely agitated, complaining that her psychiatrist was having intercourse with her through the light bulb over her bed. She was hospitalized and went into remission in a few weeks.
>
> She then wanted to continue outpatient treatment with the same psychiatrist, who also worked a half day a week in an aftercare program. At a joint meeting of the inpatient and aftercare staff, it was decided to offer her a 10-minute visit with the psychiatrist every 2 weeks to monitor her medications and write her prescriptions. At the same time she agreed to participate in the recreation activities and group therapy of the aftercare program.
>
> Now, 5 years later, she is doing well. The one-to-one relationship with the psychiatrist that had produced what was believed to be a transference psychosis was sufficiently diluted by the less frequent, brief visits and her participation in the aftercare program.

It may help prevent the patient's transference from becoming too intense if the therapist is a bit more open about his or her life than he or she would be with less disturbed patients. For example, transference concerns may prompt the patient to ask about the therapist's personal life. Unlike in the treatment of less disturbed patients, psychotic patients may be helped to be more comfortable in treatment if they know whether the therapist is married, has children, and so forth. The resident can feel free to tell the patient anything that is a matter of public record—the sort of thing one would tell an acquaintance at a cocktail party—but more personal matters should remain private. When declining to answer a patient's personal question, it is important to empathize with the patient's wish to know the answer and then to explain that refusing to answer is necessary to protect the therapeutic endeavor.

Emotional Reactions to the Patient

Clinicians interested in working with chronically psychotic patients will inevitably experience frustration, exasperation, and impatience. At times they will be tempted to scold patients for their refusal to face the truth; at other times they may feel caught up in the demoralization and hopelessness that afflicts chronically mentally ill patients so much of the time.

Clinicians also may feel inadequate or guilty as their patients complain about their failure to improve. In response the clinicians may feel against their better judgment that they should do something, such as prescribe more (or different) medication. As noted in Chapter 6, and as seen below in the case of Ms. DeBarry, however, medication prescribed to make the clinician feel better is undesirable not only because it leads to excessive use of medication but also because it prevents the clinician and the patient from addressing and dealing with the underlying frustrations that are troubling both of them:

Ms. DeBarry (continued from p. 109)

During the course of treatment, Ms. DeBarry frequently attacks Dr. Lyon for not knowing enough about psychopharmacology. "I bet if I were seeing a different doctor I wouldn't be so depressed! I need a new antidepressant!" At first, these comments make Dr. Lyon feel inadequate, defensive, and angry, but gradually he learns to distinguish affective shifts due to her illness from the sad feelings that are realistically appropriate for her situation. Consequently, he resists being baited into an unproductive argument about medicine and instead focuses on Ms. DeBarry's feelings, as by saying, "It sounds like you're having a rough day. Let's talk about how you feel."

If the clinician's negative feelings are not carefully observed and monitored, they can adversely affect his or her judgment and interventions. The exasperated clinician may become irritated and demanding with the patient, giving ultimatums and insisting that the patient immediately overcome resistance to treatment. The demoralized clinician may convey a feeling of hopelessness to a patient who is already discouraged and near despair. A useful rule of thumb is that whenever you feel you are fed up, and the patient is being willful or deliberately obstinate and should be told, in no uncertain terms, to "cut it out," it is best to take time to examine your feelings before taking action. Discussing these feelings with a senior supervisor can be helpful; a careful and disciplined perspective on the course and direction of treatment helps to counter the clinician's frustration and impatience.

Maintaining Therapeutic Optimism

The clinician needs to maintain a realistic sense of therapeutic optimism: a conviction that the situation is not hopeless but that the patient can battle his or her illness, however prolonged and difficult the struggle. Chronic patients are usually demoralized and tend to think it is hopeless to try to struggle toward normal function. Much of the early years of their treatment is devoted to dealing with the inevitable despair they suffer as they face the fact of chronic disabling illness. Because progress is often slow and punctuated by repeated setbacks, it is easy to slip into agreement with the patient that the situation is hopeless and that pain and disappointment are the only fruits of continuing efforts.

The problem for both therapist and patient is accepting the fact that the therapeutic process takes years and that most patients improve by almost imperceptible increments. In practice, the clinician often sits through many hours during which the patient complains about hopelessness and the therapist's efforts are dismissed as pointless and ineffective. It is almost always a mistake to take such criticism at face value. The patient is usually expressing genuine frustration and despair, as in the following example, but is also testing the clinician to see if the clinician is merely going through the motions or whether he or she does in fact expect ultimate improvement:

> Ms. Grant, a 25-year-old depressed woman with chronic schizophrenia, often comes to therapy full of despair. After listing all of her defects and deficits, she insists that there is little point in continuing treatment, because her case is clearly hopeless:
>
> > MS. GRANT: I'm just a fat, ugly, emotional cripple. I'm a failure and no good at anything. Therapy is just a waste of time for me.
> >
> > THERAPIST: Do you really mean that?
> >
> > MS. G.: Yes.
> >
> > THERAPIST: Then why do you keep coming to see me?
> >
> > MS. G. [*genuinely alarmed*]: Oh my God! I don't mean I want to stop seeing you—that would put me back in the hospital for sure!

In this episode the therapist misses the point of Ms. Grant's complaints. She is not threatening to terminate treatment, but rather probing to see if the therapist shares her despair and frustration. The therapist needs to continue to counsel patience and remind Ms. Grant that the work is expected to proceed slowly.

One way for the clinician to maintain hope is to keep the focus on a longitudinal perspective. Progress may be imperceptible over a period of months, but noticeable over 5 or 10 years. Looking over the patient's chart or setting up a case conference may be a useful strategy for reviewing the long-term picture. For many patients, increasing frequency and duration of periods of stability may represent significant progress, even if the patient's baseline functioning does not change.

Disruptions in Treatment

Because psychotic patients have such difficulty adapting to significant change, a therapist's absences can be particularly stressful and anxiety provoking. As inpatient units are well aware, each summer there are a flurry of admissions directly related to therapists' absences, as is seen in the following case:

> Ms. Atkinson, a 28-year-old single woman, had a 7-year history of chronic schizophrenia. She was making good progress in treatment, her symptoms were adequately controlled by antipsychotic medication, and she made good use of her weekly psychotherapy sessions.
>
> In her third year of treatment her therapist was hospitalized with pneumonia. A colleague called each of his patients, explained that the clinician was ill, and offered to meet with each patient to help deal with the separation. Ms. Atkinson, however, refused to see the covering clinician, and, although she continued to take her medication, she became progressively more withdrawn.
>
> When her therapist returned to work, Ms. Atkinson attended the first session in a severely delusional state, insisting that her therapist had "died and been resurrected." She required 3 weeks of hospitalization before she was able to resume outpatient treatment.

To help a patient cope adequately with these breaks in treatment, the patient, if at all possible, needs to be informed about absences well in advance and to have explicit coverage arrangements. This may mean that the family members should also be told of the dates of the vacation and the coverage arrangements. For patients who are marginally compensated, scheduled meetings with the covering clinician may be needed. Furthermore, unless there is a good reason not to, it is probably helpful to tell the patient who asks where the therapist will be going on vacation so that the patient can "locate" him or her in the world and feel a continuing sense of connection during his or her absence.

Beginning clinicians often believe, incorrectly, that if they handle their vacation "properly," the patient will not decompensate. This belief may lead to undue guilt for the therapist and undue pressure on the patient to discuss feelings that he or she may be adamantly denying. In fact, many psychotic patients will decompensate around vacations no matter what the therapist does, and it may take years of therapy before absences will be tolerated. Some patients habitually decompensate during the vacation, while others save their decompensation for afterward, when seeing the therapist again stimulates feelings of anger and abandonment.

Termination

Termination is an especially distressing event for the chronically mentally ill patient. Even patients who do well seldom achieve a complete termination from treatment; instead, their need for regular treatment diminishes so that they can schedule meetings at greater intervals and can regulate their own medication between meetings. Ultimately, patients may be able to schedule meetings only when issues or symptoms require assistance. Over time, the relationship with the clinician grows more relaxed and comfortable as a result of the long history of successful collaboration between the two.

Unfortunately, the realities of training programs and clinic procedures make premature and repeated changes of clinician commonplace in outpatient programs serving chronically psychotic patients. Because each change of clinician interferes with treatment, a patient who has to endure several such changes is receiving care that is far short of the optimum.

Residents who work with chronic patients during the short-term tenure of the residency may react to anticipation of termination by feeling defeated before they start. If these feelings are shared by the patient, they become self-fulfilling negative prophecies. In order to combat these feelings, the following guidelines are advisable:

1. Residents should restrict their psychotherapeutic involvement with chronic patients to a manageable number of patients with whom they can make a commitment of at least 1 year, and preferably 2 years.
2. The resident should inform patient and family, at the outset, of the maximum length of treatment in the residency program, while reserving in his or her own mind the possibility, if it exists, of seeing the patient privately after training is over.

3. Much can be accomplished in 1 to 3 years of treatment. Even just maintaining stability can help the patient to achieve progress that will not be completely lost even if the patient decompensates temporarily after termination and transfer.
4. The resident can set attainable goals, such as achieving a successful long-term medication regimen, shifting family structure to facilitate stability and improvement, having the patient begin to attend a day program, facilitating the patient's attachment to another clinician(s), and conveying a sense of hope and success.
5. The resident can continually reinforce the patient's contribution to the success of the relationship and emphasize the patient's ability to use his or her skills to succeed in relationships with future clinicians.
6. The resident needs to allow the patient to discuss feelings of sadness, loss, anger, and abandonment, even though these feelings are hard to hear and engender in the resident guilt and the wish to deny his or her termination.
7. When the reality of residency rotation requires a shorter-term contact, the resident should restrict his or her role to that of a member of the treatment team, and encourage the patient's therapeutic connection with more permanent team members.

Transfers

About 3 months prior to termination, the resident needs to actively arrange transfer of the patient to a new therapist, preferably a permanent staff member. The patient's feelings about termination, his or her resistances to transfer, and the wish to drop out of treatment all need to be worked with, although many patients will simply be unable to verbalize such feelings.

Residents should anticipate acting out and decompensation before, during, and/or after the actual transfer. This behavior is generally unavoidable, and, in some cases, an early, planned hospitalization may be a useful intervention for effecting successful transfer. The ability of the patient to request additional help in this phase can be interpreted as a sign of strength.

In addition to helping the patient express his or her concerns and frustrations, the resident can help the patient cope with the transition to a new clinician by discussing the matter well in advance, by informing the patient of the new clinician's gender and name, and, if at all possible, by arranging at least one meeting between the patient and the new therapist before the transition. These issues of termination and transfer are illustrated in the case of Mr. Maddox:

Thomas Maddox (continued from p. 108)

When Dr. Wilcox began working with Mr. Maddox, he informed the patient and his family that he would be leaving in 2 years, at the end of his training. To the family, this seemed a long way off. During the course of treatment (described in Chapter 5), the therapist achieved regulation of Mr. Maddox's medication with depot administration; education of the family to reduce the pressure for quick results; and involvement of Mr. Maddox in a day program and in vocational rehabilitation.

Now, during the course of Dr. Wilcox's termination, Mr. Maddox not unexpectedly stops coming in for his shots and begins to decompensate. With the help of the family, Dr. Wilcox admits him to the hospital, where he is stabilized and connects with a new, long-term therapist. On discharge he is able to return to day treatment, where his attachment helps to cushion the pain of transitioning to the new therapist. Ultimately, he is able to continue to progress in his social and vocational rehabilitation.

8

Involving the Family in Treatment

Matthew Jermyn (continued from p. 101)

Mr. Jermyn is to be discharged from the hospital. Dr. Transome knows that as Mr. Jermyn's therapist, he will have to maintain contact with the family. Mr. Jermyn's parents are interested in treatment only in relation to Matthew; they are not looking for "family therapy" and would resist being referred to a separate family therapist. But how should Dr. Transome go about working with the parents as well as with Matthew?

Basic Structure of Treatment

When working with families of chronically mentally ill patients, the beginning clinician is well advised not to adhere to any preconceived notions about what "family therapy" is or should be. Just as with individual patients, the therapist needs to approach each family with flexibility so as to adapt the structure of the treatment to the family's particular needs. Moreover, the clinician needs to continually reevaluate the structure of the treatment and to be ready to change the structure as the needs of the family and the goals of the treatment evolve. Some of the questions the resident may ask about the specific structure of treatment are discussed below.

Who Is Included?

In working with chronic patients and their families, the resident will frequently want to try to simultaneously engage all significant family members, to maintain an individual relationship with the patient, and to provide opportunities for the family to discuss the patient in his or her absence—all in an hour a week or less. It helps to begin this process by discussing these issues explicitly with the patient alone, the family alone, and with everyone together.

Matthew Jermyn (continued from p. 119)

Dr. Transome sets up a meeting with Mr. Jermyn and his parents, specifically to discuss the structure of outpatient treatment. First, he meets with Matthew alone:

> DR. TRANSOME: I plan to meet with you and your parents every week. It's important for you and me to continue our individual time, but I also need to spend time alone with your parents, and with all of you together. Since I only have one hour a week, how would you feel about our meeting for a session every other week and dividing the intervening sessions between you and your parents?
>
> MR. JERMYN: As long as we meet every week, I guess it's O.K. for you to spend some time with my family. But I don't like them talking to you about me behind my back. I want to be there when you meet with them.
>
> DR. T.: We can do it that way sometimes, but I think it's in your interest for your family to have a chance to talk to me alone so I can help them to help you better. They'll feel freer to talk with me that way, just as you do. I'll make sure that you are kept informed of anything that comes up that you need to know about. Can we give it a try?
>
> MR. J.: Well . . . O.K.

Dr. Transome then speaks with the family alone, to decide how often they will meet and who should come. In order to make it clear to the family that they are being involved in treatment as collaborators, not as patients, Dr. Transome opens the meeting with the following comment:

> Your involvement as collaborators in your son's treatment is very important. This does not mean that you caused the illness. But because you play such an important role in Matthew's life, any strategy for rehabilitation that does not involve you will probably not succeed.

Mr. Jermyn's parents agree, and although they wanted weekly contact, they compromise on a half-session every other week. Although Matthew's adult siblings are not interested in being included, Dr.

Transome makes clear that they will always be welcome, if later they wish to come. Finally, Dr. Transome meets with Mr. Jermyn and his parents together to go over the agreed-upon structure and to explain that periodically they will all meet together.

The arrangement Dr. Transome devises for Matthew's parents is only one of many possibilities. With some chronic patients, the family requires full sessions, and the patient only brief contact; with others, all significant family members need to be regularly included. In any case, the therapist needs to convey an accepting attitude toward whoever comes in, and not interpret missed sessions or missing family members. If family members are to view themselves as allies in treatment, not as the subject of treatment, they must participate in their own style without criticism or disapproval by the therapist.

When and Where Are Sessions to Be Held?

Although the frequency of meetings with the family can vary according to the case, most families require relatively frequent meetings in order to sustain a treatment relationship or to attain treatment goals. For some families, however, monthly or even quarterly meetings may suffice. Often, an initial series of relatively frequent meetings may establish a treatment relationship that can be sustained by regular but less frequent contact.

Even the location of family sessions may require flexibility. Home visits demonstrate the willingness of the therapist to extend himself or herself to meet the family on their own terms, and help the family to feel more like collaborators and less like patients. Home visits can also help to engage resistant or disorganized families, and provide insights into family functioning not otherwise possible.

Carol Oliva

Carol Oliva, a 28-year-old woman with schizophrenia, lives at home with her elderly parents. Her mother, who was at one time diagnosed as having a schizotypal disorder, has befuddled a series of family workers because of her confused and disorganized speech and her seeming inability to understand her daughter's illness.

Ms. Oliva's new doctor decides to engage the family through weekly home visits. The doctor observes that despite the mother's disorganized speech, she is competent as a homemaker. The doctor's ability to support her homemaking and mothering helps her to be more receptive to his guidance about her daughter's illness.

How Should the Therapist Interact With the Family?

Many of the guidelines that were described for individual treatment also apply to working with the family. The major focus of family sessions early in treatment is to make the family comfortable with you. Families of chronically mentally ill patients feel guilty and overwhelmed, and often they have been attacked and criticized by mental health professionals. Therefore, the clinician tries to join with the family in a supportive, nonconfrontational, friendly manner, at the same time maintaining a professional demeanor.

Joining with families often means participating in casual conversation or social rituals to put families at ease, as in the following examples:

Carol Oliva (continued from p. 121)

During home visits to the family of Ms. Oliva, the schizophrenic young woman mentioned earlier, a routine develops in which the doctor sits with the family in the kitchen while the mother serves coffee and toast. The "sessions" begin with casual conversation about the events of the week before moving on to discussion of problems.

Mr. Parker (continued from p. 108)

Sessions with the anxious, overinvolved parents of Mr. Parker, the young man with schizophrenia whose case was discussed briefly in Chapter 7, always begins by the resident's putting the parents at ease:

RESIDENT: So how are you both this week?

FATHER: O.K. It hasn't been a bad week.

MOTHER: I'm real worried about Larry; he's been very nervous.

RESIDENT: Yeah, I know. I'm also concerned about how you have been?

MOTHER: Not too bad. I try to get my mind off it.

RESIDENT: How's your job?

MOTHER: Getting busy, but I'm doing well.

RESIDENT: That's great. You need to be involved with something that makes you feel good. And [*to father*] how's the produce business?

FATHER: Business is awful. No one's buying onions this time of year.

RESIDENT: Why not?

[*The father launches into discussion of his business.*]

The resident's clear interest in developing her alliance with the parents sets a friendly, informal tone that helps them to be willing to make difficult changes in how they deal with their son.

Even when a family is being outrageous, confrontational, angry, or demanding, as in the case of Mr. Quinn's family, consistent support is essential to maintain the alliance:

Mr. Quinn (continued from p. 105)

The mother of Mr. Quinn, the young man with schizophrenia described in Chapter 7, is frustrated with her role as sole support of her family in the face of her husband's chronic unemployment. She constantly vents her frustration and dissatisfaction with everyone, and, in particular, she is highly critical of her son's ongoing disability. Because the therapist refuses to join her in attacking the patient, she begins each session with a lengthy complaint about the lack of progress in therapy. The resident is challenged to cope with his frustration and anger and to find ways of being supportive:

> MOTHER: As usual, my son isn't doing anything at all. He's just lazy! Every time he tries anything, he claims his "voices" bother him. What a bunch of hooey! And all you doctors do is pump him full of medicine. You know, I don't think it does him a bit of good.
>
> M.D. [*resisting the urge to argue*]: It must be tough for you to be the one carrying the whole load.
>
> MOTHER: Yeah. I'm the only one around here who does anything! How on earth are we going to get our son moving?
>
> M.D.: Is he working on that behavior contract we set up?
>
> MOTHER: He does a few things, but it's like nothing. He needs a job. You're too easy on him.
>
> M.D.: I know it's slow, but a few weeks ago he wasn't doing anything. This disease is terribly frustrating, and progress is so slow.
>
> MOTHER: Well, I feel there's hardly any progress at all, though I suppose he is a bit better.

What Is the Content of Sessions?

Residents need to resist the temptation to explore feelings, ask probing questions, make interpretations, and so forth. Because families of mentally ill patients do not define themselves as patients, it is important in maintaining an alliance with the family not to treat them as patients, not to use family systems jargon, and not to make an interpretation unless it can be done in a way that does not put the family on the defensive.

While meeting with Ms. Oliva and her parents (see above), the resident observed that whenever the parents disagreed about how to help their daughter, Ms. Oliva said something outrageous to refocus attention on herself. In this situation a *formal* "system" interpretation would cast blame on the family system for the patient's illness and is likely to provoke a guilty or defensive response:

> RESIDENT: Have you noticed how your daughter uses her symptoms to try to control arguments between the two of you? Maybe her illness functions to prevent marital difficulty?

Instead, an *informal* "system" interpretation keeps the session moving without implying blame:

> RESIDENT: Gee, Carol, you certainly don't like to see your parents fight.
>
> CAROL: What do you mean?
>
> RESIDENT: When they were disagreeing about how to help you with your illness, you did a great job of getting them to stop by talking about the devil. You make a great peacemaker.
>
> ALL: Laughter.
>
> RESIDENT: Now, let's keep working on helping Mom and Dad agree on how to help Carol. I know Carol gets nervous when she feels things aren't clear.

A more focused comment, not a systems interpretation, also keeps the session on track:

> RESIDENT: I know you're upset about your parents' disagreement, but it's important for us all to work this problem through. Let's see if we can stay with the topic and come up with a solution.

Interpretations are usually unnecessary if not directly related to the task at hand.

The focus for family work needs to concentrate on attainable, not overambitious, goals that are relevant to the management and rehabilitation of the patient's illness. Instead of trying to change the family, the resident tries to help the family cope with the illness and support the patient; most treatment contracts do not sanction intervention in family problems not specifically related to the patient.

We will now examine some specific goals of family involvement in treatment, using case examples to illustrate how the resident might work toward these goals.

Goals of Family Involvement in Treatment

Support

The importance of building a supportive relationship between the family and the resident cannot be overemphasized. In many families, simply introducing a supportive physician into the family system can have a significant impact on the family's ability to manage the patient, and consequently on the course of the illness. The Oliva family illustrates this point:

Carol Oliva (continued from p. 122)

Ms. Oliva, the younger of two daughters, had been close to her mother throughout her childhood. Her mother, as noted earlier, was a schizotypal, histrionic woman who responded to emotional stress with rambling, tangentiality, and tearfulness. The patient's father was a controlled and rational but angry man who viewed both his wife and the mental health system as incompetent.

Both were highly invested in their daughter and had taken care of her from the onset of her illness at age 21 through a rocky and downhill course that culminated in her admission to the state hospital when they felt unable to care for her anymore. Through this period, the mother had burned out a succession of family therapists with her denial of her daughter's illness, her lack of focus, and her inability to form an alliance, all related to her fear that she was to blame for the illness. The father, by contrast, had made gradual progress in understanding the nature of his daughter's illness and the need for the parents to play a collaborative role in Ms. Oliva's recovery. He could see how his wife's inability to accept and work with the illness made it difficult to cope with her.

After Ms. Oliva had spent a year in the hospital, the staff asked a psychiatric resident in the parents' hometown to work with them. The resident met with the couple without the patient every 2 weeks for the next year, patiently reiterating the concept that Ms. Oliva had an illness and that the mother was not to blame. The mother eventually began to trust the resident enough to agree.

At this point, a meeting was held with the daughter, on the state hospital ward, in which the family presented their newly united front to their daughter. In the meeting the mother spontaneously said: "Listen to the doctor. He's right. You do have an illness and you have to learn to accept it. It took me a long time to trust the doctor and admit that, but now I do, and we want you to do it too."

Six months later, Ms. Oliva returned home. With continued weekly support and periodic home visits from the resident, the parents are better able to manage her, and she has remained out of the state hospital for over 2 years.

Education

An important aspect of family work is continuing education of the family about mental illness and its course and management. Families—and patients—need frequent review and repetition to overcome their denial and their resistance to facing the painful reality of the disease. Families and patients may also need reeducation as new issues or new data emerge during the course of treatment.

Reinforcement of Medication Compliance

Because families are often the most powerful agents available to enforce or reinforce medication compliance (see Chapter 6), they require ongoing education about its importance. Many patients who refuse medication are covertly supported in their refusal by a key family member who does not believe that medicine is necessary or is reluctant to "drug" the patient. By working with the family to overcome denial and resistance, the resident often can help develop a united front that can enforce ongoing compliance. These principles also apply to the role of the family in fostering support for and compliance with the psychosocial aspects of the treatment plan.

As in the case of the Jermyns, families may need to make medication compliance a condition of the patient's remaining at home. In most instances, however, families can enforce this rule—with the help of the psychiatrist—simply by a show of force, without needing to resort to such an extreme measure as eviction:

Mr. Parker (continued from p. 122)

After several years of medication compliance and stability, Mr. Parker stops his trifluoperazine and soon becomes paranoid. During their regular meeting with Mr. Parker's psychiatrist, the patient's parents say that their son's behavior is so intolerable that he will have to leave home unless they can be assured of medication compliance. When Mr. Parker joins the meeting, he is confronted with his noncompliance and is offered a choice between starting intramuscular fluphenazine as an outpatient or being hospitalized to restart trifluoperazine:

MR. PARKER: What if I don't do it?

PARENTS: Then you can't stay at home until you do!

MR. P.: But I have nowhere else to go!

M.D.: So, you have to make a choice.

Mr. Parker then agrees to enter the hospital to restart trifluoperazine and to continue to take the medication after he is discharged.

Family Empowerment

With the Patient

One of the biggest problems facing families who live with mentally ill relatives is how to deal with the patients' intimidating or demanding behavior. Family members may attempt to set limits but do not know how to enforce them effectively. Families are often advised to enforce limits by putting the patient out of the house, but they consider this step too harsh, too dangerous, or too extreme. Consequently, they may unwittingly begin to let the patient run the show, leading to a chaotic and overburdened household. A major focus of ongoing family treatment can be helping families develop strategies for setting limits and enforcing them.

One technique is to help the parents use money, cigarettes, soda, and so forth, as contingencies for empowerment.

A mother, whose son is chronically schizophrenic, complains that her son never bathes or cleans his room:

MOTHER: All he does is sit and smoke.

M.D.: And where does he get the cigarettes?

MOTHER: Well, I give him three packs a day.

M.D.: And what does he do in return?

MOTHER: Oh. I see what you mean.

With the System

Empowerment of the family within the larger mental health system is often a goal of ongoing family treatment. Families may need the resident to be their advocate, to help them obtain access to resources, and to help them to validate their needs and concerns. Families often have great difficulty being "heard" by the system, as in the following example:

A 32-year-old schizophrenic woman is living with her parents, as she has done for her entire life, except for one brief period when she had tried to live alone but became blatantly psychotic and had to be hospitalized. The patient resists medications, and her parents find monitoring her compliance to be a constant challenge. It is difficult for them to be assertive and to take charge of their household by setting reasonable limits on the patient. They also feel increasingly that they should have a life of their own apart from taking care of their daughter.

Finally, with much hesitation, the parents ask their daughter's psychiatrist to hospitalize her for 2 weeks while they take an overseas trip. The psychiatrist recognizes that the parents are becoming "burned out" and that, without a period of respite, they might totally withdraw from the patient. Despite the fact that the patient attends a day treatment center as well as participates in regular psychiatric treatment, the psychiatrist knows that she is not at all ready for a permanent out-of-home placement and separation from the parents. The psychiatrist therefore arranges for her to be placed in a temporary "crisis house" for the 2-week period. The parents return refreshed, ready to take up where they had left off with the care of their daughter.

Working Toward the Next Step

Rehabilitation

An important function of ongoing family treatment is to help the family develop appropriate strategies for encouraging the patient to participate in a program of social or vocational rehabilitation. Family members often will prematurely push the patient to go to work, and then get frustrated or give up entirely if the patient cannot hold a job. Such families require considerable education about the need for the patient to proceed slowly. Families also need information about available rehabilitation programs and how to identify which program(s) will be most helpful. Once the appropriate program is identified, the next step for the family is to determine how to get the patient to go. Families often need to be encouraged to let patients proceed at their own pace, and to resist the urge to push or nag.

Carol Oliva (continued from p. 125)

When Ms. Oliva returns home from the state hospital, her parents are concerned about her lack of activities. Ms. Oliva complains of loneliness and speaks often of missing her friends at the state hospital. Nevertheless, she is unwilling to go to day treatment, because she is frightened of meeting new people and wants to avoid other sick people.

In the early months of Ms. Oliva's return, many family sessions focus on helping her parents to be patient and not to nag their daughter into attending a program or to push her to think about work. The resident lets Ms. Oliva know that when she is ready, she can begin to attend a social club; after 6 months, she decides to try it. Although at first she is frightened and negative, she is also motivated to be with her peers. Gradually, at her own pace, she begins to feel more comfortable and in 6 more months works her way up to full-time participation in the prevocational clubhouse program.

Some patients seem to get stuck at home, never wanting to go out or to attend any programs. When families accept this behavior, the therapist may be tempted to struggle with them to satisfy his or her need to see results. Acceptance of the current equilibrium in the family system, however, is the only way to proceed.

In most families the parents push or nag "stuck" patients, who may then, in turn, dig in their heels in more determined resistance. This is often enacted through superficial compliance with parental demands followed by passive-aggressive sabotage:

***Mr. Quinn** (continued from p. 123)*

Mr. Quinn's mother prods him to join a day program that he does not want to attend. He resents her pressure, but cannot openly defy her. He attends the day program regularly for a week but then gradually begins to come late and miss sessions. When confronted by program staff and his increasingly frustrated parents, Mr. Quinn angrily threatens to stop his medicine and refuses to return to the program.

Separation

A common issue in ongoing family treatment is when to encourage the family to move the patient out and when to encourage the patient to leave. Families often develop relationships with patients that are labeled "enmeshed," "overinvolved," or "symbiotic"; these negative labels can be used to conclude that the patient needs a "parentectomy." This line of reasoning is usually incorrect, and efforts to attempt to force premature separation generally backfire. Chronically mentally ill patients and their families need to approach separation slowly so as to be assured that in each case the patient is capable of handling the separation and that the necessary supports are available.

The following example illustrates successful and unsuccessful approaches to this problem:

Andrew Barton, a 25-year-old man with schizophrenia, has an "enmeshed" relationship with his mother; whenever he tries to live apart from her, one or the other becomes psychotic. Yet when they live together, the relationship is chaotic and they continually quarrel. Two years earlier, neighbors called the police several times because of the loudness of their fights. After these episodes, the patient's psychiatrist strongly recommended separation and placement of the patient in a halfway house, and both patient and mother reluctantly went along with the plan.

Living alone, the mother has become lonely and depressed, while the patient not only misses his mother but feels guilty about leaving her alone. After 6 weeks the patient becomes psychotic; after a brief hospitalization he returns to his mother, and the relationship continues as it had before.

Dr. Carter, a new psychiatrist, takes over the case. He considers separating the patient from his mother and discusses the situation with both parties separately and then sees the two of them together. Although mother and son say that they will do whatever the psychiatrist recommends, he emphasizes that while he can clarify their options for them, it is ultimately their decision. After several difficult, and at times stormy, meetings, mother and son decide to continue living together, and Dr. Carter, as he had promised, supports their decision.

Therapy continues weekly with the patient and monthly with the mother. The patient is enrolled in a day treatment center and progresses to a sheltered vocational workshop, while the mother is encouraged to become more involved in her church and to develop a limited social life. Four years later, the patient tentatively brings up the idea of moving to a halfway house. Although both he and his mother are ambivalent about this move, they decide after another 6 months to go ahead with it. This is a difficult time for both, but they are able to survive the separation.

The kind of close but ambivalent parent-child ties exemplified by the previous case can meet many needs, and giving these ties up may make a bad situation worse. Except under extreme conditions, therefore, the therapist's role is to clarify options rather than to exert pressure.

Contracting

Working with families to develop individualized behavior contracts in the home is an important task of family treatment and can be useful both in helping the patient to take responsible action and in helping the family to structure their expectations more concretely. Behavior contracts allow defined rewards and restrictions to replace inconsistent praise and criticism. The contracting process is illustrated in the following case example:

Rosalie Johnson, a 34-year-old chronically schizophrenic woman, complains of feeling empty, bored, and unproductive. Her mother reports that she had demonstrated artistic talent before the onset of her illness, but that now she rarely draws. Ms. Johnson's occasional flurries of activity are inconsistent and unscheduled; she rarely cooks, does housework, or assists with the care of her 10-year-old son. She fills up her empty time mooning about her ex-husband and dreaming of going to Hollywood.

After several months of developing an alliance with the family and helping the patient's mother to stop struggling to control her daughter, the psychiatrist believes that it might be time to address Ms. Johnson's negative symptoms:

M.D.: Would you like some help in getting things done?

MS. JOHNSON: I guess so.

M.D.: We then have to set up a program in your home to help you get going. With your kind of mental illness, it's hard to be productive; but when you are not productive, you feel empty. The only way out is to start making progress, one step at a time. Do you see what I mean?

MS. J.: Yeah, I guess so.

M.D.: We'll start slowly because we want you to feel successful. Let's start with a regular schedule each day for a constructive activity. The schedule is important because following a regular routine helps you to get organized. You can start with as little time as you can manage comfortably and then build up from there. It could be 5 minutes a day, 15 minutes, an hour, and so forth—whatever you feel you can do. It's better to do 15 minutes a day on schedule, regardless of how you feel at the time, than to do 3 hours one day and the next day nothing. Does that make sense?

MS. J. AND HER MOTHER: Yes.

M.D.: What would you like to do?

MS. J. [*after some discussion with her mother*]: Sewing children's clothes?

M.D.: How long can you manage each day? 15 minutes? 30? 1 hour?

MS. J.: An hour.

M.D.: Are you sure that's not too much?

MS. J.: I don't think so.

M.D.: Well, keep a record of how much you do. If it's less than an hour a day, we can change the schedule.

MS. J.: O.K.

M.D.: Now we need a specific time each day, and which days.

[*Ms. J. selects 10:30 to 11:30* A.M. *Monday through Friday, and the resident writes down the assignment and sets up an appointment for the next week.*]

More elaborate and comprehensive contracts can be developed as well (see Appendix E). Most texts on behavior therapy contain examples of contracts that can be used by the resident.

Working on Family Dynamics

At times, ongoing family treatment focuses gently on unhelpful patterns of family interaction that seem to precipitate recurrent difficulties for both patient and family. Because most family members are already burdened with feelings of guilt and failure, any interventions are best framed positively and supportively so as not to add to that burden.

Fostering Appropriate Detachment

A family's need to change the patient often leads to frustration. Although this feeling may begin with love and concern, it can result in anger and criticism when the patient repeatedly fails and the family does not see progress. In such instances, family treatment can focus on helping the family not to try so hard to fix, control, or improve the situation. Family members may need encouragement to lead their own lives as much as possible and to seek gratification and support from sources other than the patient, as in the following example:

Martin Douglas is a 28-year-old single man with a long history of drug and alcohol abuse and schizophrenia. His parents were both alcoholic, and as a child he developed a passive-aggressive style for coping with his rage without risking his parents' uncontrolled anger. At present, his mother is dead, and his father has 10 years of sobriety. Mr. Douglas lives with his father, has 2 years of sobriety himself, and is well maintained on medication. However, his continued passive-aggressiveness is a major problem. His father, who is overinvolved, angry, and controlling, continually pushes him to hold a job and work in the house. Mr. Douglas superficially complies, and then sabotages himself, leaving his father to bail him out. When the father becomes enraged, the son feels resentful and angry, and the cycle continues.

The focus in family treatment is on encouraging the father to back off and helping him to take responsibility for himself:

FATHER: He drives me crazy. I tell him to set the alarm to get to work on time, but he doesn't do it. He stays in bed, and then I have to yell at him to get up.

RESIDENT [*to Martin*]: How do you feel about this?

MR. DOUGLAS [*shrugging*]: I don't know. I don't like it, I guess.

RESIDENT: Why don't you get up?

MR. D. [*shrugging*]: I don't want to go to work.

RESIDENT: So why do you?

MR. D.: I need the money.

FATHER [*interrupting*]: If he doesn't have money, I have to pay for everything.

RESIDENT: You have to?

FATHER: Well, what else am I supposed to do?

RESIDENT: You might consider backing off. As it is, you may be making things too easy for Martin and too hard for yourself. By fighting with Martin, you let yourself be the bad guy, and Martin doesn't have to take responsibility for making his own choices. Right, Martin?

MR. D. [*enjoying his father's discomfiture*]: Yeah.

RESIDENT: So that means it's up to you to decide if you want to work or if you want to be on welfare.

MR. D.: Well, I guess I would really rather work.

RESIDENT [*to father*]: It's easier for both of you to let Martin figure out what he's going to do. You deserve to give yourself a break.

FATHER: You know, I think you're absolutely right. I do too much for him; I've got to let go.

Reducing Anger and Criticism

Strategies for reducing anger usually start with understanding the family member's anger as an indirect plea for more support. Support of the angry relative by the resident may allow the anger to be refocused on safer targets and provide room for more positive regard toward the patient, as in the following case:

Ms. Lester is a socially and politically prominent 55-year-old woman whose 30-year-old son was diagnosed 5 years ago as having chronic undifferentiated schizophrenia. Ms. Lester has denied that her son is ill and has explained his behavior as resulting from stress at college, an unhappy love affair, nutritional deficiencies, and/or inept handling by physicians and psychiatrists. She harasses her son's psychiatrist and does not want her son to take maintenance medication even though her son says that he feels better when he is taking it.

The psychiatrist meets frequently with Ms. Lester. As she gets to know him better, Ms. Lester intensifies her angry comments and reproaches him for the "many failures of psychiatry." She paradoxically denies that her son is mentally ill and, at the same time, berates the psychiatrist for not finding an effective treatment for him. She also warned him that she intends to complain to the Department of Mental Health about him. At this point, the psychiatrist is tempted to tell Ms. Lester that her anger and disappointment are so great that he does not think that he can work effectively with her and her son, and to recommend that her son obtain psychiatric treatment elsewhere.

The psychiatrist recognizes, however, that this response would be acting out his own angry feelings, and instead responds:

RESIDENT: I agree with you. It is a tragedy that psychiatry cannot do a better job of treating your son, and I wish I could do much more for him—and for you. I'm sure that if I were in your shoes I too would complain to the Department of Mental Health. In fact, letters like that might help to let the politicians know that they need to spend more money on programs and research for the mentally ill.

MS. LESTER [*surprised, yet pleased*]: Well, I never expected you to agree with me. But you're certainly right that those politicians don't care about the little people. My poor son suffers so; he tries so hard, and no one cares.

In this instance, the physician joins the mother's anger, redirects it to a safe target, and uses it to continue to build the alliance. The more supported the mother feels, the more empathy she displays for her son.

Conclusions

Involving the family in the ongoing treatment of people with chronic mental illness can permit a wide variety of valuable and powerful interventions that can facilitate the patient's improvement. Family treatment is also rewarding and enjoyable for the resident. Once the resident masters the technique of joining instead of struggling with the family, he or she can become a significant part of the total family process of adapting to the major catastrophe of mental illness, and can appreciate the value of his or her unique contribution to the family's well-being and survival.

9

Using Community Treatment Programs

Susan Foster

Susan Foster, a 25-year-old single woman with a bipolar disorder, was doing well on lithium and thioridazine maintenance, attending weekly psychotherapy, and working full time. She was doing so well that her thioridazine was discontinued, whereupon she experienced a devastating manic episode, despite adequate lithium levels. She was hospitalized nearly 5 months before she could be restabilized on lithium, carbamazepine, and thioridazine. During that time, she lost her job, her apartment, and much of her self-confidence. Even now, after she has stabilized, she feels unable to concentrate adequately or to function independently.

Rather than return to work and to independent living, she agrees, with the help of her therapist, to live in a cooperative apartment and attend a community day treatment program. In her psychotherapy, she works to increase her self-esteem and to overcome her sense of failure and hopelessness. Gradually, in the day treatment program, she is able to socialize more actively, build her confidence through increasingly responsible tasks, and ask for support more directly.

After about a year, she feels ready to make the transition to a supported work program. Her goal is to return to competitive employment in a less demanding job, with the support of her therapist and the program counselors. Four months later, she is working. She continues to live in the co-op apartment, but is looking forward to eventual independent living. Even after "graduating" from all program supports, she plans to remain in weekly psychotherapy with her psychiatrist.

Ms. Foster's case illustrates the successful use of community treatment resources in the stabilization and eventual rehabilitation of an individual with a chronic, disabling mental illness. For Ms. Foster, these resources included community residential placement, day treatment, and vocational rehabilitation services, in addition to individual psychotherapy and pharmacotherapy.

The range of systems and treatment programs that are used by chronically mentally ill individuals and families, the needs that different types of programs address, and a methodology for assessing the network of services available to particular patients in each community system of care have been presented in Chapter 4 (see also Appendix C). In Chapter 5 we described the use of community resources in treatment planning, specifically in the cases of Mr. Maddox, Mr. Jermyn, Ms. DeBarry, and Ms. Hogarth. In this chapter we will focus on issues that arise with the implementation of the use of community programs in the course of ongoing treatment.

Most residents find that success stories like that of Ms. Foster are rare. In Ms. Foster's case, her needs were matched both by her willingness and her capacity to seek out services to address those needs, and by the availability of suitable resources and programs at the times she needed them. In the "real world," however, residents' efforts to incorporate community treatment programs—or, at times, hospital treatment—into their work with chronically mentally ill patients are often frustrated by formidable barriers that must be addressed and resolved in the treatment process for the plan to proceed successfully. Failure to address these barriers as a natural and expectable phase of treatment can result in burnout for both the resident and the patient.

The major barriers to the use of community treatment resources are as follows:

- Disagreements about the patient's needs
- Unwillingness or inability of patient or family to accept referral or to follow through
- Inability of patient to use needed services
- Improper timing of referrals
- Treatment team conflicts
- Lack of available resources

In most cases, more than one of these barriers—and in some cases, all of them—will need to be addressed.

For example, in the case of Mr. Maddox (described in Chapter 5), the resident's initial recommendation that the patient needed more social support would have been opposed both by the patient, whose focus was mostly on symptom relief, and by the family, who wanted more individual contact with a psychiatrist and a focus on Mr. Maddox's returning to work. Even had Mr. Maddox agreed that he needed more social contact, he would have resisted referral to a day program or social club, based on his previous bad experiences with groups. And even had he been persuaded to "try it," his paranoia would have made him unable to attend successfully. Consequently, an initial attempt by the resident to pursue a social club referral would have been made at an inappropriate time and thus would have backfired.

Progress in treatment, therefore, is not measured by the speed with which patients can be cajoled into attending community programs. Residents may feel pressured, both by the glib assessments of others ("Your patient definitely needs a day program") and by the residents' uncertainty about managing a case alone to pursue referrals and placements prematurely.

There is no satisfactory shortcut that will bypass patiently working with patient, family, and community resources to achieve a collaborative plan. Any such plan must address the barriers listed above through the following steps:

1. Develop agreement about needs.
2. Develop willingness to accept referral.
3. Assess capacity to participate in the treatment program.
4. Address treatment team issues.
5. Implement a plan for accessing limited resources.

Agreeing on Needs

Some patients will not accept the need for the additional support of a day program until they have failed to make it on their own:

> Ms. Cutler, a 26-year-old woman who has been slowly decompensating for 2 years, has her first full-blown psychotic break when her husband announces plans for divorce. During her first hospitalization, her psychosis clears rapidly with medication, and her husband agrees to stay. She nevertheless remains anxious and somewhat disorganized, and resists acknowledging the seriousness of her illness, in part because of her fear of turning out like her mother, who was chronically schizophrenic. She refuses day treatment, insisting that she will return home to find work. Within weeks of discharge, she becomes overwhelmed with anxiety and suicidal feelings and has to be readmitted. Then, reluctantly acknowledging that she needs more support before returning to work, Ms. Cutler accepts a referral to day treatment.

At times, the resident may have to wait patiently through a series of failures and discouragements before a patient can acknowledge a need for help. In the following example, the resident allowed a patient and family to pursue a plan that he knew would not work in order to prepare them to accept his recommendation to proceed more slowly:

> The parents of Robert Harkins, a chronically delusional homebound patient with schizophrenia, insist that their son needs a referral to a vocational program, believing that having a job would "drive those crazy thoughts out of his head." The patient agrees with his parents, but when asked to define his vocational goals and plans, he becomes disorganized and grandiose, rambling on about becoming a stockbroker and earning "millions." The resident's attempts to explain to the family about the patient's level of disability and the slow process of rehabilitation are met with angry resistance. Only after the resident agrees to make the referral, and the family is told by the vocational program that the patient is currently incapable of using vocational resources, can they agree to participate in a more limited treatment program.

Developing a Willingness to Accept a Referral

Although patients and families may agree with the resident about the need for a referral, they may be unable to accept it, as in the case of Mr. Parker:

Mr. Parker (continued from p. 127)

Mr. Parker, the 29-year-old schizophrenic man living with his parents who was described in the previous two chapters, complains of being bored and lonely and of having too little to do. Suggestions of referral to day treatment or vocational programs are met with strong resistance: he does not want to be involved with "crazy" people. Although he says he wants a "real" job, he takes no steps to look for one. Mr. Parker's parents constantly nag and criticize him about his laziness but at the same time make life easy for him by providing generous supplies of cigarettes, soda, rides, clothes, and so forth.

The resident supports Mr. Parker's right to choose how to engage in treatment and to resist being nagged, and explores and gently confronts the patient's resistance to engaging in rehabilitation. At the same time, the parents are encouraged to set clearer limits and contingencies for their financial support.

It takes over a year before the parents are able to say that funds for cigarettes, soda, and recreation will be stopped unless the patient attends a day treatment or vocational program. The patient then decides to accept a referral.

The success of Mr. Parker's treatment plan depends not only on the family's coercion but on the resident's alliance with the patient. The resident first determines that the patient is in fact capable of performing in such a program, and then works through the patient's resistance to the rehabilitation process.

Patients resist referrals to treatment resources for many reasons, some of which are listed in Table 9–1.

Mr. Parker (continued from above)

Mr. Parker feels that both the doctor and his family should make things easy for him, and believes that his father owes him a job in the family business. He has little self-confidence and is angry that he is expected to work despite his illness. The resident accepts Mr. Parker's anger at his family's control, while pointing out that the effort Mr. Parker is making to try to change them makes him the ultimate loser. She also offers hope, stating that she believes that he is more capable than he thinks, and that he is selling himself short by waiting for his parents to give everything to him.

Many patients and families need patient and repeated education about the realistic problems of rehabilitation. Thus, patients who object to the boredom of day treatment, as in the following case, may need to be confronted with their difficulty adhering to any schedule and with the reality that a more challenging program could be even harder to follow consistently:

Mr. McGraw, a 35-year-old man with schizophrenia, resists attending his clubhouse program, saying he wants a job. Although he claims the

Table 9–1. Reasons for resisting referral to community treatment programs

Denial or minimization of illness
Lack of information about the rehabilitation process
Anger at being ill and needing to "work" to get better
Despair and hopelessness
Self-disgust and lack of confidence because of illness
Belief that the family should solve the problem
Wish to be dependent and remain disabled
Magical restorative fantasies

clubhouse is too easy, he often leaves after becoming overwhelmed and anxious:

> MR. McGraw: That clubhouse is too easy for me, so I get bored and just leave. I really should be working.
>
> RESIDENT: You do a great job of covering up your disability; it must be painful for you to admit how hard that clubhouse program is for you. The staff there tell me that you leave when you get overwhelmed and anxious.
>
> MR. McG. [*quietly*]: Yeah, I guess so, but I don't know why.
>
> RESIDENT: People with schizophrenia have a hard time handling stress and changes. To get better you have to take it slowly but consistently. Going to the clubhouse one afternoon a week and asking them to help you stay is better in the long run than going several days in a row and then staying away for a month.

Assessing the Patient's Capacity to Participate

As Mr. McGraw's case illustrates, residents need to be careful not to urge referrals before the patient can participate.

Mr. Quinn (continued from p. 129)

The resident wants Mr. Quinn to attend a full day treatment program in order to improve his socialization and provide structured time away from his critical mother. The resident, however, overestimates Mr. Quinn's ability to tolerate a full day of social interaction without becoming overwhelmed. On the third day, Mr. Quinn begins hearing more voices and leaves the program. He is eventually able to succeed at a less demanding program, which requires him to attend only three mornings per week.

Some patients may not be able to fit into any program, either because there are none available that will meet their needs or because of the realistic limitations of their chronic mental illness.

Mr. Maddox (see Chapters 5 and 7), for example, was too paranoid to tolerate the social club programs that would have addressed his loneliness and isolation. It took 2 years before consistent medication and a supportive treatment alliance reduced his paranoia enough to permit him to participate in a social club. During this period, the resident tolerated listening to Mr. Maddox talk about his painful loneliness, realizing that there was little he could do.

At times, the patient's level of incapacity requires prolonged state hospitalization, as in the following example:

> Harold Mullins, a chronically mentally ill 22-year-old man with a learning disability, has been placed by his mother in a group home because of his persistent rages and suicidal behavior. He does well at first, but as his relationships in the program intensify, he becomes extremely sensitive to fantasied rejection by the other patients, culminating in a serious suicide attempt by the patient. Several hospitalizations followed by residential placements lead ultimately to the same result. The treatment team finally realizes that even though the patient is not floridly psychotic, he cannot be maintained safely in a community residence, and state hospital admission is arranged. After 6 months, his behavior control and internalized ability to deal with affect have improved enough to permit transition to an on-grounds dormitory setting.

Addressing Treatment Team Issues

The resident's need to collaborate with the treatment team was discussed in some detail in Chapter 4, where we observed that referring a patient to a community program requires both resident and patient to develop a relationship with the staff of that program. A resident who has been treating a patient and family for a year or more may find it difficult to have to share the case with other clinicians, some of whom may have different clinical perspectives, and none of whom have the same kind of alliance with the patient. In such referrals the resident needs to walk a fine line between, on the one hand, advocating vigorously for the program to meet the patient's needs and, on the other, detaching enough to allow the patient to adjust to the program's requirements.

Matthew Jermyn (continued from p. 121)

> After a year of treatment, including consistent medication compliance, Mr. Jermyn has improved to the extent that Dr. Transome considers a referral to day treatment. Although Mr. Jermyn is much less floridly psychotic, he still looks odd, and under stress he occasionally makes bizarre statements. He has been attending a social drop-in center fairly regularly and doing well, but his participation is not at all structured. Dr. Transome, unsure whether Mr. Jermyn would meet the day program's requirements, arranges to visit the program with him, as described in the vignette in Chapter 4 (p. 65).
>
> In the interview at the day program, Mr. Jermyn's presentation is marginal. However, Dr. Transome pleads for the staff to give him a chance, describing the progress Mr. Jermyn has made in the last year

and how hard he has worked in therapy. Dr. Transome also agrees to be available for team meetings, case conferences, and consultations.

Because of his psychiatrist's involvement, Mr. Jermyn is provisionally accepted by the day treatment program. Dr. Transome, in relaying this news, emphasizes to Mr. Jermyn the importance of consistent attendance: "This program will be a challenge for you. The expectations to attend regularly are new. If you can do it, great, but if you can't, you may need to drop the program and wait till you're a little stronger." Mr. Jermyn replies that although he is nervous, he feels ready and thinks he can succeed.

Dr. Transome's willingness to participate in case conferences with other members of the treatment team is vitally important. Inevitably residents feel burdened by the extra time demands of case conferences when their patients are using community programs. Participation in these treatment team meetings, however, is perhaps even more important in the long run than meeting with the patient; lack of coordination within the treatment team can often render all therapeutic efforts fruitless.

Facing the Lack of Resources

The inadequacy of treatment resources for chronically mentally ill patients in many areas is frustrating, as in the following example:

Mary Hogarth (continued from p. 109)

Dr. Lincoln believes that Ms. Hogarth needs an integrated program where her therapy, medication, and vocational workshop can all be coordinated in one location. His frustration is evident as he complains to the community mental health center director about the lack of such programs.

The director replies, "If you are frustrated, imagine how the Hogarths feel. But we can't abandon them because we feel frustrated. The lack of resources is a fact of life, at least for now; we need to see it as a clinical challenge. How do we help the Hogarths—or any other patients and their families—make the best use of the resources that are available?"

Reframing the absence of resources as a clinical problem helps to keep the resident from joining the patient in feeling helpless and stuck by inadequacies in the system. The resident can acknowledge that resources are limited, but although this limitation may delay the patient's recovery, it does not make it impossible. Instead, it challenges the resident to help the patient to develop skills that are likely to promote success.

Mr. Quinn (continued from p. 140)

Mr. Quinn has repeatedly said that he wants to move into a community residence. His psychiatrist notes that while this might be a good plan, there are no available placements for patients who already have a place to live.

He points out the options to Mr. Quinn: "We can certainly put in an application for a halfway house, but as long as you're living at home you probably can't get in. I'm sorry about it, but we just have to face it and work on helping you to make it at home. We can do this by getting you involved in more programs and activities outside the house, such as the social club, and by helping you to be less sensitive to your mother's criticism."

In another situation, the resident uses the existence of a waiting list as an opportunity to prepare the patient more thoroughly:

Ms. DeBarry (continued from p. 112)

Ms. DeBarry has been pushing Dr. Lyon for referral to a supported work program. When she goes for an interview, she is accepted but is told that she will have to wait 4 months before she can begin. She becomes furious and storms out of the interview.

When Ms. DeBarry reports this to Dr. Lyon, bemoaning the inadequacy of the system and vowing to find work on her own, Dr. Lyon confronts her immediately:

> You are quick to fly into a rage when something doesn't go your way. We've talked before about how your anger hides your difficulty coping with your disability; as we both know, you're scared to death of working, and suddenly you can't wait a few months more to go to work. I think this 4-month wait may be a blessing in disguise. Finding that you can live with uncertainty and anxiety without bolting will be excellent preparation for dealing with the kind of frustration you will encounter when you get a job.

10

Dual Diagnosis

Joseph Taraminia

Only a few hours after admitting Mary Hogarth to the inpatient unit (see Chapter 1), Dr. Holt receives another call from the emergency room. Joseph Taraminia has once again been brought in by the police. The triage nurse relays the major elements of Mr. Taraminia's history: He is 24-years-old, living with his mother, with a 6-year history of schizophrenia and a 10-year history of polysubstance abuse, primarily alcohol, marijuana, and cocaine. He has a history of five previous state hospital admissions, ranging from 3 days to 12 weeks; he has been arrested many times for fighting, loitering, and making threats; and he has had even more admissions to the county detox center. He takes medication only intermittently and attends a psychiatric day treatment program sporadically.

Tonight, Mr. Taraminia had a fight with his mother and apparently stormed out of the house. He has evidently been drinking and may have been smoking crack as well. He was picked up by the police after he was seen staggering in the street, muttering about a conspiracy involving "the FBI, the CIA, and the Papacy."

Dr. Holt knows that most young chronically mentally ill patients have coexisting substance abuse and that these patients are notorious for being difficult. The alcohol and drugs make the mental illness worse. And yet the drug problem cannot be treated because of the mental illness.

Some of the issues involved with dealing with dual-diagnosis patients are the subject of this chapter.

Recognition of the Problem

Joseph Taraminia (continued from p. 145)

When Mr. Taraminia is interviewed by Dr. Holt, he denies drinking or taking any drugs, stating that he is just upset because his mother threw him out of the house after an argument over playing the radio too loudly. He says that if Dr. Holt would just call his mother and ask for her to take him in, she would. He smokes and sips a soda continuously.

As Dr. Holt gets farther into the interview, Mr. Taraminia becomes more agitated, angry, and paranoid, much as he was described by the emergency room staff when they called her. The patient mumbles incoherently but threateningly about the CIA and FBI, and seems to slur his words at times.

Dr. Holt is tempted to take his denial of substance use at face value; because he is clearly psychotic, she considers that to be his "primary" diagnosis. She recalls, however, that substance intoxication can mimic acute psychosis, particularly in patients with underlying chronic mental illness, so she decides to order a blood alcohol level and a urine toxic screen. The blood alcohol comes back nearly three times the legal limit for intoxication, yet Mr. Taraminia is wide awake. Dr. Holt is surprised by the extent of Mr. Taraminia's tolerance for alcohol.

As this case illustrates, identification of dual-diagnosis patients often requires a high index of suspicion that allows the resident to go beyond the patient's denial or minimization to seek other sources of data, such as toxic screens or family caregivers' reports.

Once the presence of substance use is confirmed, the next problem is making a diagnosis. If the patient is unknown to the treatment system, it might not be possible either to diagnose a major mental illness or to assess the extent of his or her substance use disorder until he or she has been sober for as long as 2 weeks, so as to observe whether the psychosis clears completely without antipsychotic medication. If the psychosis clears, the patient might then be assumed provisionally to have a primary substance use disorder and a toxic psychosis. On the other hand, if the psychosis does not clear, or, as in the case of Mr. Taraminia, the patient has a well-documented history of mental illness, he or she could be assumed to have two primary illnesses—a primary mental illness and a primary substance use disorder—each requiring specific and simultaneous treatment.

But which substance use disorder does Mr. Taraminia have? The DSM-III-R diagnostic criteria for psychoactive substance dependence and abuse disorders are listed in Tables 10–1 and 10–2, respectively. These criteria can be applied to chronically mentally ill patients as follows.

Table 10–1. DSM-III-R diagnostic criteria for psychoactive substance dependence

A. At least three of the following:

1. Substance often taken in larger amounts or over a longer period than the person intended.
2. Persistent desire or one or more unsuccessful efforts to cut down or control substance use.
3. A great deal of time spent in activities necessary to get the substance (e.g., theft), in taking the substance (e.g., chain smoking), or in recovering from its effects.
4. Frequent intoxication or withdrawal symptoms when expected to fulfill major role obligations at work, school, or home . . . , or when substance use is physically hazardous (e.g., drives when intoxicated).
5. Important social, occupational, or recreational activities given up or reduced because of substance use.
6. Continued substance use despite knowledge of having a persistent or recurrent social, psychological, or physical problem that is caused or exacerbated by the use of the substance . . .
7. Marked tolerance: need for markedly increased amounts of the substance (i.e., at least a 50% increase) in order to achieve intoxication or desired effect, or markedly diminished effect with continued use of the same amount.
8. Characteristic withdrawal symptoms.[a]
9. Substance often taken to relieve or avoid withdrawal symptoms.[a]

B. Some symptoms of the disturbance have persisted for at least 1 month, or have occurred repeatedly over a longer period of time.

[a]May not apply to cannabis, hallucinogens, or phencyclidine (PCP).
Source. Reprinted from American Psychiatric Association: *Diagnostic and Statistical Manual of Mental Disorders,* 3rd Edition, Revised. Washington, DC, American Psychiatric Association, 1987, pp. 167–168. Copyright 1987, American Psychiatric Association. Used with permission.

Table 10–2. DSM-III-R diagnostic criteria for psychoactive substance abuse

A. A maladaptive pattern of psychoactive substance use indicated by at least one of the following:

   1. Continued use despite knowledge of having a persistent or recurrent social, occupational, psychological, or physical problem that is caused or exacerbated by use of the psychoactive substance.

   2. Recurrent use in situations in which use is physically hazardous (e.g., driving while intoxicated).

B. Some symptoms of the disturbance have persisted for at least 1 month, or have occurred repeatedly over a longer period of time.

C. [The patient has] never met the criteria for psychoactive substance dependence for this substance.

Source. Reprinted from *American Psychiatric Association: Diagnostic and Statistical Manual of Mental Disorders,* 3rd Edition, Revised. Washington, DC, American Psychiatric Association, 1987, p. 169. Copyright 1987, American Psychiatric Association. Used with permission.

Substance *abuse* is defined as any persistent harmful use of substances, where harm may be defined as making a concomitant illness worse. Because all psychoactive substances, including caffeine and nicotine, can 1) increase psychiatric symptoms, 2) interfere with the effectiveness of antipsychotic agents, 3) increase emotional instability and acting out, and 4) interfere with successful adaptation to mental illness, it follows that all persistent psychoactive substance use in chronically mentally ill individuals can meet the criteria for substance abuse disorder and should be treated as such.

The diagnostic criteria for substance dependence require the presence of harmful consequences such as the exacerbation of psychosis as well as loss of job or residence, arrest, and so forth, and lack of control of use as evidenced by bingeing or intoxication, with or without clear-cut tolerance or withdrawal. Based on Mr. Taraminia's history of arrests and relapses due to intoxication, his frequent lack of control of use, and his high tolerance to alcohol, Dr. Holt can confidently make a diagnosis of alcohol (as well as caffeine and nicotine) dependence, in addition to schizophrenia.

Establishing Safety

Mr. Taraminia's intoxication and agitation present an immediate problem for Dr. Holt. Her assessment cannot be completed accurately while the patient is intoxicated, yet he is clearly too unstable to be discharged from the emergency room. His obvious psychosis prevents him from being admitted to an ordinary detox unit, but his high alcohol level prevents him from being accepted for admission by the state hospital. Consequently, in order to ensure Mr. Taraminia's safety prior to establishing a relationship, a diagnosis, or a treatment plan, Dr. Holt needs to hold him for 12 to 24 hours until he becomes sober enough to permit evaluation of his baseline mental status; in this case it was possible for Mr. Taraminia to be held in the emergency room. Once Mr. Taraminia is sober, his ability to maintain safe behavior and his need for containment can be reassessed.

Engaging and Assessing Patient and Family

Joseph Taraminia (continued from p. 146)

Next morning, when Dr. Holt returns to the emergency room to reevaluate Mr. Taraminia, she finds a different person. Mr. Taraminia is sober and calm. His affect is a bit flat and his thinking somewhat loose and concrete, but he is no longer overtly psychotic. He seems to have little recollection of how disturbed he had been the night before, and is anxious to return home. His mother has come down to pick him up.

Dr. Holt sees no reason to assume that anything has changed, despite Mr. Taraminia's glib promise that he has "learned his lesson" and will stop drinking and taking drugs. Her negative feelings about persons who abuse alcohol and other drugs and her resentment of the time she has spent with Mr. Taraminia to no apparent avail make her want just to let him go and let him be someone else's problem. Although she knows she will not act on these feelings, she does not know what else to do. When she calls Mr. Taraminia's day program for more information, staff members report that he continues to deny the severity of the problem, and they plead with Dr. Holt to do what she can to break through the denial.

Dr. Holt knows that denial and minimization are as much a part of the disease of alcoholism as they are a part of mental illness. She realizes that Mr. Taraminia's lying is part of his disease and that her best chance of breaking through his denial is to begin a process of engagement. So she starts by saying the following:

DR. HOLT: You know, Mr. Taraminia, the day center staff is concerned about your marijuana and alcohol use.

MR. TARAMINIA [*sullen and instantly on guard*]: So?

DR. H.: What's going on from your viewpoint?

MR. T. [*irritated*]: Nothing. They just think I shouldn't drink. But I don't really have a problem.

DR. H. [*empathetically*]: So you think the staff doesn't understand?

MR. T. [*smiling*]: Yeah!

DR. H. [*with continued empathy*]: It must be really hard to have so many people trying to run your life.

MR. T. [*more open*]: Yeah, I don't know what their problem is. All my friends drink and drug a little. I only do it when I go out with them, so I don't see why they have to make such a big deal about it. They're threatening to drop me from the program if I don't stop.

DR. H.: You're really in a rough spot. But I guess that you need to make your own decisions about drugs and alcohol.

MR. T. [*relaxing*]: Yeah.

DR. H.: So tell me, what do you really think? In your opinion, have you ever had a problem with drugs? How much have you used?

MR. T.: Well, I used to smoke a lot of grass . . . [*hastily*] but not anymore.

DR. H.: How much is a lot?

MR. T.: I used to smoke a couple of joints a day from when I was 15.

DR. H. [*neutral and friendly*]: That much? What about now?

MR. T.: Oh, only a couple of times a week. [*His manner seems less than honest.*]

DR. H. [*not in a confronting manner*]: How about alcohol and other drugs?

MR. T.: I only drink with my friends once a week or so. I haven't used other drugs.

DR. H. [*laughing*]: Never?

MR. T.: Oh, well, maybe speed a few times, or cocaine—just once. I did take LSD a few years ago.

DR. H.: So you don't feel you have a problem?

MR. T.: No.

DR. H.: Do you want to hear what I think?

MR. T. [*curious, but guarded*]: I don't know.

DR. H.: Well, it's up to you.

MR. T. [*more in control*]: O.K.

DR. H.: My biggest concern is you. I want to help you to make your decision about your drug and alcohol use based on your knowing what's best for you, given that you have a mental illness.

In this interview, Dr. Holt avoids a direct struggle with Mr. Taraminia about his substance use and begins an alliance based on supporting the patient's autonomy and his right to make his own decisions. Dr. Holt knows that Mr. Taraminia is still minimizing the extent of his use, but she avoids directly challenging him because she knows he will just stop answering.

At this point in the interview, Dr. Holt might continue her exploration of Mr. Taraminia's substance use in a neutral, noncritical manner. (Some of the questions that might be asked, including some questions specific for dual-diagnosis patients, are presented in Appendix F, which is derived from the Michigan Alcohol Screening Test.) Dr. Holt might take this opportunity to inform Mr. Taraminia of her views about the harmful effects of substance use on patients with schizophrenia, and of her opinion that he may be an alcoholic. She must be careful, however, not to lecture. She needs to continue to give him a sense of control over what he wants to hear and an opportunity to express his point of view. The goal is to educate him into making better decisions about his substance use, not to browbeat him into submission.

Joseph Taraminia (continued from above)

Later, Dr. Holt returns to a discussion of what happened the night before. Mr. Taraminia's first response is to project blame onto his mother:

MR. TARAMINIA: My mother was really furious at me last night.

DR. HOLT: Furious?

MR. T.: Just because I had a little to drink.

DR. H.: Tell me about it.

MR. T.: Well, I borrowed some money and bought a few beers, and my mother got uptight about it.

DR. H.: How many beers?

MR. T. [*hastily*]: About 12 . . . but it was over 8 hours.

DR. H.: Anything else?

MR. T.: A little rum, I guess.

DR. H. [*still in a nonconfronting manner*]: And how did your mother find out?

MR. T.: I have no idea. I wasn't staggering or anything . . . well, maybe a little. I think she heard me get sick.

DR. H.: You got sick?

MR. T.: Yeah, I threw up . . . then I drank some more . . . so I couldn't have been that drunk.

DR. H.: Did you keep going until all the beer was gone?

MR. T.: Yeah.

DR. H.: How come you didn't get some more?

MR. T.: I had no more money . . . anyway, she started yelling at me, and I started yelling back a little. And then she called the cops!

DR. H. [*making her move*]: Do you think this might indicate a problem?

MR. T.: No way. It's just my mother gets so upset.

DR. H.: Well let's take a look. You tell me you borrow money to drink, you drink two six-packs, you get noticeably drunk, you get so sick you wake up your mother, you keep drinking anyway till all the money and beer are gone, and you create a family disturbance. I wouldn't be surprised that you'd do it again tonight if you had the money.

MR. T.: Probably . . . well, no . . . I don't know.

DR. H.: I think there's a lot of evidence for your drinking getting you in trouble. Maybe you need to keep an open mind about whether you really do have a problem.

MR. T.: Well, maybe. But the real reason I drink is because of my mental illness. I get so nervous! And drinking makes me feel better. Maybe if you gave me some Valium?

DR. H.: What other medication are you on?

MR. T.: Well, the clinic psychiatrist wants me to take Prolixin shots, but I don't like that. I mean . . . when I go to AA, they say, "Don't get hooked on chemicals." I don't want to be dependent on the stuff. Maybe if I just stay sober, my craziness will go away.

DR. H.: It sounds like you're trying to figure out what your "real" problem is. Are you *really* an alcoholic—and all your craziness will go away if you get sober, or are you *really* a schizophrenic—and you only drink because you're mentally ill? Do you want to know what I think your *real* problems are?

MR. T.: Sure, Why not?

DR. H.: You really have two illnesses—you have both schizophrenia and alcoholism. Each one makes the other one worse, and you need treatment for both!

MR. T.: Maybe . . . maybe so . . . but . . . what can I do about it?

In this vignette, Mr. Taraminia illustrates many facets of the denial of the dual-diagnosis patient: blaming family members, medication, and other patients for his drinking; and using "shifting denial"—that is, using mental illness as an excuse not to get help for mental illness. In this instance, Dr. Holt's empathic manner succeeds in temporarily breaking through some of the denial.

Joseph Taraminia (continued from p. 152)

Before Dr. Holt can develop a treatment plan, however, she needs to engage Mr. Taraminia's mother. Dr. Holt finds that Ms. Taraminia, like many family members of substance-abusing and dual-diagnosis patients, is both furious at her son and unable to let go:

> MS. TARAMINIA: He's all I've got left since my husband died! He needs me. I mean, with this schizophrenia or whatever, he can't take care of himself—now can he? And he's really a nice boy—really—except when he drinks. I could kill him! I pour the liquor down the drain—and he just gets more. Why can't he just drink sociably? And he lies! He promises, promises . . . and then boom! There he goes again. I keep saying, "Get help. Get help," but does he listen? No way. Not him. Just like his father, may he rest in peace. Drank himself to death, he did. But at least he wasn't violent.
>
> DR. HOLT: Do you think your son is alcoholic?
>
> MS. T.: Alcoholic. What's an alcoholic? Maybe he is, maybe he isn't. I mean, he doesn't drink every day does he?
>
> DR. H.: It sounds like things have been really rough living with him.
>
> MS. T. [*tearful*]: You should only know. It's such a trial, I don't know how I survive. But what can I do? They say, "Put him out!" But I could never do that. He's my son! And I'm all alone! Do you think I should put him out?
>
> DR. H. [*thinking that she certainly would, but she answers empathically rather than giving advice*]: I can imagine how you feel. You love him and you worry about him. But what do you think we should do? We can't make him stop drinking.
>
> MS. T.: I don't know what to do. If only he would go for help.

At this point, Dr. Holt might gather more information about Mr. Taraminia's substance use (see the questions in Appendix F) and assess the history of substance use in the family, as well as previous efforts at treatment. Dr. Holt might also reinforce the mother's need for help in her own right, not only for relief but also for her to acquire more education about alcoholism and learn strategies to stop enabling her son and to begin to confront him.

Once Dr. Holt feels that Ms. Taraminia's anger has subsided, she decides to try to have a three-way meeting. She encourages Ms. Taraminia to tell her son how much she loves him and hates to see him hurting himself, and to tell him she can't make him do anything, but it would mean much to her if he would get help. Mr. Taraminia, softened by the rapport he had built with Dr. Holt, agrees.

In this vignette, Dr. Holt has successfully used empathy to engage both Mr. Taraminia and his mother. She takes the stance with both of them that no one has the power to make Mr. Taraminia stop drinking, and uses the mother's concern as a tool to encourage her son to be willing to seek help. The next problem Dr. Holt faces is assessing system resources for the dual-diagnosis patient, and then designing a treatment plan.

Assessing the System

Based on Mr. Taraminia's history of out-of-control behavior, his continuing medication noncompliance, and his tendency to decompensate under stress, Dr. Holt believes that inpatient treatment is the best first step in Mr. Taraminia's recovery. Although many non–mentally ill drug-addicted and alcoholic persons can get sober simply by attending AA or NA, dual-diagnosis patients find it more difficult. Special support and education are usually needed, on an inpatient unit and/or in a structured outpatient setting, to help the patient learn how to distinguish between symptoms of mental illness and addiction, and how to engage in a program of recovery or rehabilitation for each illness. Dr. Holt is also aware that once inpatient treatment is completed, Mr. Taraminia is likely to need ongoing structure in the outpatient setting to maintain stability of both illnesses through medication compliance and sobriety:

Joseph Taraminia (continued from p. 153)

Dr. Holt consults her resource manual and finds that in her area there are alcohol and drug abuse detoxification programs, residential rehabilitation programs, and drug-free and drug-assisted (Antabuse or methadone) outpatient programs. But she also knows that most of these programs hesitate to take on patients with severe mental illness. Her senior resident tells her that he has worked out an arrangement with one residential program that involves 24-hour backup by the psychiatric emergency service with its dual-diagnosis patients in case of crisis, which has made this program less reluctant to accept such people. However, the program only takes patients who have completed an inpatient detoxification and/or rehabilitation program.

When she calls the 12-step alcohol rehabilitation program, Dr. Holt senses an unstated but distinct disapproval of accepting anyone who is taking any medication, even an antipsychotic. She tries to convey tactfully that she understands that AA nationally accepts such people, but the admitting person is clearly skeptical, saying that Mr. Taraminia's need for individual attention and structure could not be met at AA. Dr. Holt then tries a widely publicized drug-free inpatient substance abuse program, where the admissions person describes a highly confrontational approach, which Dr. Holt is convinced Mr. Taraminia cannot tolerate. So she turns to her university hospital services, but the inpatient staff is openly hostile toward persons who abuse alcohol and other drugs. Also, there is no addiction treatment component on the unit or AA meeting in the hospital, and the staff is untrained in substance abuse treatment.

Dr. Holt searches her resource manual for an "integrated" or "hybrid" program, in which the staff is trained in treatment and rehabilitation of both psychiatric and substance use disorders. There are none in the immediate area, but after several phone calls to outlying hospitals, she locates a suburban general hospital with a combined psychiatry and addiction unit that will accept Mr. Taraminia's insurance.

Dr. Holt is still concerned about Mr. Taraminia's housing, because there are few community residences available and none specifically for dual-diagnosis patients. As noted earlier, one addiction halfway house will accept patients on medication, but only if they are fairly high functioning, and she is not sure Mr. Taraminia will qualify. In any case, he is likely to return home.

Dr. Holt begins to think that the answer is not to abandon the day program, but to build upon it. She calls the general hospital's consultation-liaison substance abuse counselor, who is himself a recovering alcoholic. She describes her problem with Mr. Taraminia's treatment and asks the counselor if he would be willing to help establish a recovery support group and/or an AA meeting at the day program, because she knows of several other day treatment members with similar problems. The counselor agrees to cooperate, and Dr. Holt volunteers to contact the day program director to set up a planning meeting, provided Mr. Taraminia is agreeable.

Dr. Holt's experience is not unique; "dual diagnosis" programs are often hard to find. Nevertheless, with energy and creativity, treatment resources can frequently be located or developed. Locating resources is only part of the problem, however. Treatment planning can go nowhere unless the patient is motivated to cooperate.

Developing a Treatment Plan

Joseph Taraminia (continued from p. 155)

When Dr. Holt returns to the treatment area after finishing her phone calls, she finds Mr. Taraminia urgently whispering to his mother. They both look up guiltily as Dr. Holt walks in. She senses something has changed, but she nevertheless begins to present the plan she has developed of hospital treatment followed by day treatment with a recovery support group and AA. Mr. Taraminia interrupts:

> MR. TARAMINIA: I'm not going to a hospital! Right, ma? [*Dr. Holt looks at Ms. Taraminia.*]
>
> MS. TARAMINIA: Joseph has promised he will stop drinking. His uncle will take him to AA. He says he's really serious this time. [*Ms. Taraminia seems as if she is trying hard to convince herself.*] I said I'd give him one more chance.

Dr. Holt is furious, thinking that she has done all that work for nothing and that Mr. Taraminia has just wrapped his mother around his finger. But Dr. Holt controls herself and decides that the only solution is to give them enough rope:

> DR. HOLT: I'm glad you two have worked out a plan. As you know, I suspect that Joseph will need more than just AA to stop drinking, but it's O.K. with me if you want to give it a try. Now, what happens if he does drink again?
>
> MR. T.: Oh, don't worry, Doc!
>
> DR. H.: I'm not worried, but I think your mother is worried.
>
> MS. T. [*white faced*]: I can't take much more . . .
>
> MR. T.: Oh come on, Mom! I'll be fine.
>
> DR. H.: Let me make a suggestion. Mr. Taraminia—you're sure you'll be O.K., right?
>
> MR. T.: Right!
>
> DR. H.: How about if I set up a regular meeting with you and your mother to monitor your progress. If you stay sober, great! But we'll sign a contract that if you get drunk again, you won't be able to stay at home until you go through a treatment program.
>
> MS. T.: Yeah! That's a good plan—and I know your uncle Bob will agree. You sign that contract, Joseph.
>
> MR. T.: Ma, come on. I'll be fine!
>
> MS. T.: Sign it!
>
> MR. T.: Oh, all right.

In this vignette, Dr. Holt once again confronts the reality that a treatment plan for dealing with dual diagnosis depends on engaging patients with empathy and awaiting the opportunity for confrontation by significant others (e.g., family members, treatment providers, or police) that may push the patient into accepting treatment.

Meanwhile, Dr. Holt needs to maintain a stance of empathic detachment: she can help Mr. Taraminia if he is willing, but she is responsible neither for his sobriety nor for protecting him from the consequences of his continued drinking. If he gets in trouble, that is his problem, and it may provide further impetus for him to seek treatment. In this frame of mind, Dr. Holt proposes a contract in which she "wins" either way: either he stays sober or he enters treatment. With dual-diagnosis patients, it is much better to wait for the confrontation to develop naturally than to try to force the issue prematurely.

Joseph Taraminia (continued from p. 156)

Dr. Holt sets up an appointment for Mr. Taraminia and his mother to return in a week. She then tells the emergency room staff to notify her if he reappears sooner. Two nights later she gets a call: Mr. Taraminia's mother and his uncle, brandishing the signed contract, have brought Mr. Taraminia in drunk. The next morning, he meekly accepts hospitalization at the dual-diagnosis unit.

Ultimately, Mr. Taraminia's treatment plan will consist of the following elements:

1. Inpatient "dual diagnosis" treatment, including
    a. Detoxification from alcohol
    b. Stabilization of psychosis on depot medication
    c. Education about addiction and sobriety, and how to use AA to recover
    d. Education about schizophrenia and medication compliance, and how to use day treatment
    e. Family education and support
    f. Transition to outpatient follow-up
2. After discharge, ongoing weekly individual and family therapy with Dr. Holt, who will also function as case manager to integrate the patient's dual program
3. Continuing day treatment, including the newly developed recovery group
4. Alcoholics Anonymous daily for 3 months, then 4 to 5 times per week

Implementing a Treatment Plan

Implementing a treatment plan with dual-diagnosis patients involves individual education and therapy, working with community agencies such as AA, and working with families.

Education, Triggers, and Coping Skills

Following Mr. Taraminia's discharge, Dr. Holt helps to organize a caregivers' conference involving the addiction counselor and the day program. In the discussion, a member of the day program staff points out one of the triggers or precipitants for Mr. Taraminia's drinking: after trying, unsuccessfully, to date a female patient, he deals with his disappointment by drinking. He then comes home agitated and/or psychotic, vents his frustration at his mother, and winds up in the emergency room.

One goal of treatment, therefore, is to educate Mr. Taraminia about this pattern and help him to talk about his feelings of inadequacy and rejection, rather than drink over them. When he brings these issues up in AA and the recovery group, he is surprised to find that other alcoholic persons have similar problems. They advise him that he will be able to interact with women better after he has had a year of sobriety under his belt and that he should not try to date until then. He appears relieved by this advice.

Helping Patients to Use Alcoholics Anonymous

After 2 months of abstinence and medication compliance, Mr. Taraminia announces to Dr. Holt that he is stopping his medication. She asks why, and he replies, "People at AA tell me to stop my medicine because alcoholics shouldn't use medicine."

Dr. Holt knows of the conflicting messages between AA and psychiatry about the use of medication. So, when she first began working with Mr. Taraminia, she took time to become familiar with the AA program by attending an open meeting and by reading AA literature. She has tried to keep an open mind and think about how the program works, rather than disparaging it.

She discovered that many of the negatives she had heard about AA were stereotypes, applying to some individuals or particular AA groups but not characteristic of the program as a whole. She realized that many of the AA "steps" of recovery were also applicable to chronic mental illness: accepting your illness, needing to ask for help, not blaming yourself for your illness, getting better "one day at a time." Moreover,

"Living Sober" specifically states that AA members can take medication, and that they should listen to their physicians, not to other AA members, for medication advice. One of the women who spoke at the AA meeting that Dr. Holt attended was on lithium, spoke openly about her need for both AA and medication, and was well received.

With this background, Dr. Holt can gently confront Mr. Taraminia's attempt to use AA as a reason to stop his medication. Asking him what specifically has happened, she discovers that he had asked some of the men he met if he should take his tranquilizer, adding that he was not sure he really needed it. The response he got was predictable.

Dr. Holt observes that he is using AA as a support for his wish that he did not need medication, and that if he had made it clear that he thought he needed medication, the "people in AA" might not have objected. Dr. Holt points out that AA is where he goes for help with his alcoholism, not where he goes for advice on how to treat his schizophrenia. She then reiterates that he has two illnesses, with a specific treatment program for each.

Helping the Family System

After a few months of sobriety, Mr. Taraminia's mother tells him she thinks he is so much better he can stop "all these extra things." She needs him at home evenings, so maybe he can stop the AA meetings. Mr. Taraminia mentions this in his recovery group, and the substance abuse counselor calls Dr. Holt to report this development. Dr. Holt in turn calls the day program, which reports that Mr. Taraminia is indeed doing well but that the staff is also concerned.

Dr. Holt decides to meet with Mr. Taraminia and his mother together. She discovers that his mother is lonely at night and that she relies on her son for companionship. Also, Ms. Taraminia does not really understand alcoholism and the inability of the alcoholic person to rely solely on "willpower" to maintain sobriety; consequently, she does not appreciate the need for her son to attend AA.

Dr. Holt begins by educating Ms. Taraminia about alcoholism and then reviewing the improvement that Joseph has made. She offers to include Ms. Taraminia in regular therapy for continued support and education. Finally, she discusses the prospect of Ms. Taraminia attending Alanon, and locates a meeting that is held in the same location as one of her son's AA meetings, but in a different room. With Dr. Holt's support, Ms. Taraminia agrees to follow this plan.

Maintaining Realistic Goals

At the end of her first year of residency, Dr. Holt rotates to a service where she cannot continue to see Mr. Taraminia, and consequently she must terminate treatment with him. At the time, he was doing well.

Unfortunately, about 18 months later Dr. Holt gets a phone call from the resident in the emergency room. Mr. Taraminia is back, smelling of beer and ranting about plots against his life. The resident, Dr. Smith, summarizes the case as "hopeless," pointing out that Mr. Taraminia has been in every drug and alcohol treatment program in the area and has "failed" in every one.

Dr. Holt is tempted to agree; she is discouraged after having worked so hard 2 years earlier to find the right program for Mr. Taraminia, even tailor-making what she thought would work. Not only is he not "cured" of either condition, he seems to be no better than before. Is it time to give up?

Not necessarily. People suffering from "only" alcoholism and drug addiction or "only" chronic schizophrenia are hardly likely to recover quickly or the first time around; certainly, people with two illnesses are likely to have double trouble. Dr. Holt needs to modify her expectations, to assume slow progress, and to work toward the long rather than short haul.

After helping Dr. Smith work out another referral for Mr. Taraminia, Dr. Holt is able to feel a sense of detached concern rather than hopeless disappointment. She has not given up on Mr. Taraminia; on the other hand, however, she no longer feels personally responsible for his repeated difficulty.

Finally, as the following case illustrates, successful outcome for dual-diagnosis patients is possible, even in seemingly impossible cases, although it may take a long time before something happens to help the patient to get serious about recovery:

> Lois Delaney, a 40-year-old gay woman, has been an alcoholic and drug addicted person like her father since age 16, and has been schizophrenic since age 21. In 20 years she has had about 30 hospitalizations for violent paranoid psychotic episodes associated with medication noncompliance and substance abuse. Despite her persistent substance abuse and her verbal abusiveness when drunk or psychotic, her mother has always taken her home and has never been able to enforce limits.
>
> When Ms. Delaney's mother finds out she has terminal cancer, Ms. Delaney decompensates and is rehospitalized in the state hospital. When she is ready to leave, her mother for the first time refuses to take her home, saying, "I'm too sick now to deal with her." Because Ms. Delaney has no other options, she is in danger of remaining in the state hospital indefinitely. However, after 2 months—much longer than usual—her psychiatrist believes that mother and daughter might be

ready to compromise. With considerable support, Ms. Delaney's mother agrees to the following plan:

> Ms. Delaney could come home only if she agreed 1) to admit herself to an addiction treatment unit, and then hook up with AA; 2) to restart intramuscularly administered medication, to be given at home; and 3) to be immediately kicked out, and probably hospitalized, if she refused medication or used alcohol or drugs.

Ms. Delaney reluctantly agrees to the plan once she sees that her mother and her psychiatrist intend to collaborate to enforce the limits. After the confrontation, Ms. Delaney goes to the addiction treatment unit and begins intramuscular medication. Despite much resistance, she gradually hooks up with AA, and for the first time in her life she realizes that she can socialize without drinking.

When her mother dies 6 months later, Ms. Delaney remains sober and continues her medication, saying, "This is what my mother would have wanted." She does not decompensate.

She now lives with her aunt and uncle, who are also sober in AA. After a year of sobriety—the first year in 20 that she has had no hospitalizations—Ms. Delaney comments to her psychiatrist that AA has helped her to acknowledge her alcoholism and to feel better about herself, and thanks him for not giving up on her.

11

Treatment of Homeless Mentally Ill Persons

Joseph Drummond

Dr. Dickens is on call for the emergency room one Saturday night when he is notified that Joseph Drummond has shown up again. Mr. Drummond is homeless and is well known to the staff of the hospital emergency room. Dr. Dickens has heard about him from his fellow residents, but has never met him before.

Mr. Drummond's story is well documented in his record. Now 28 years old, he had been in his senior year at the local university when he developed schizophrenia, and consequently he never finished college. Following his initial hospitalization, he refused his parents' offer to return home, instead getting a room near the university, where he supported himself on Supplemental Security Income (SSI). He soon dropped out of psychotherapy and saw a psychiatrist only once a month for medication. He took medication inconsistently and did not request additional services.

After living in the room for 2 years, he began to develop paranoid ideas about his neighbors. He also had begun to use his SSI check to buy alcohol and had fallen behind on the rent. When the landlord approached him about the rent money, his paranoia increased, and he impulsively left the rooming house. He had no particular destination in mind, nor did he leave an address with the Social Security office so that his checks could be forwarded. He took no medications with him and began sleeping on the streets and in parks. He sometimes ate in missions, occasionally stole food, and supported himself by panhandling and begging on the periphery of the university. He spent most of his time listening to voices.

Over the past 4 years, he has become a familiar figure in the university community: filthy, unkempt, with long hair and beard, feet wrapped in rags, occasionally talking out loud to his voices. Yet he has managed to survive on the streets and has never been assaultive or suicidal. Periodically, however, he comes (or is brought by police) to the emergency room when he has had too much to drink and/or when his voices become frightening. The staff want to have as little to do with him as possible, so they give him a little medicine, call him "noncommittable," offer him help (which he invariably refuses), and send him out into the streets once he has sobered up.

This is the scenario that greets Dr. Dickens as he arrives in the emergency room. Although the sight of Mr. Drummond is so repulsive that he can barely stay in the same room, Dr. Dickens feels intrigued by the man's history, and he is somehow drawn to respond to Mr. Drummond's fear and desperation. He decides to make a serious attempt to engage Mr. Drummond.

Dr. Dickens offers Mr. Drummond a sandwich and coffee, which are eagerly accepted, and gives him some medication. Mr. Drummond relaxes somewhat, but is still guarded. Dr. Dickens speaks to him gently: "You seem to be afraid. It's hard to live on the streets, yet you are scared to ask for help. I'm worried about you—would you like my help?"

Mr. Drummond nods faintly. Dr. Dickens, sensing that Mr. Drummond cannot define what he wants or needs, says, "I'm going to admit you to the hospital. I would like to keep you in a safe place where we can give you medicine, food, and shelter, get to know you a bit, and help you to get off the streets."

Mr. Drummond looks terrified. He shakes his head vigorously in opposition and rises to leave. Meanwhile, Dr. Dickens debates whether to commit him as "gravely disabled," because he is clearly neither suicidal nor violent, and is not obviously malnourished. He decides to try a different approach: "I'm sorry that the idea of a hospital is so scary, and I don't want to force you to go if it isn't necessary, so I'll let you leave for now, but I want you to think about coming to see me as an outpatient. Otherwise, you'll be back here, and eventually you will have to go to the state hospital."

Mr. Drummond now looks even more scared, but he takes the offered appointment card, stuffs it into his pocket without looking at it, and leaves abruptly. The next day, much to Dr. Dickens's surprise, Mr. Drummond keeps the appointment. In the initial session, Mr. Drummond rambles in a disorganized way about his paranoid delusions concerning "enemies" on the street. Dr. Dickens does not challenge him and remains consistently empathic about his patient's need for safety, support, and protection. Mr. Drummond also accepts for his "nerves" a supply of perphenazine, which he begins to take daily.

By the third visit, Dr. Dickens is able to persuade Mr. Drummond to accept voluntary hospitalization. After several days of hospitalization and medication, Mr. Drummond is much less bothered by his schizophrenic symptoms. When asked why he had not arranged to receive his SSI checks or to obtain other help, he replies, "Things that would normally occur to me did not occur to me. I just could not think clearly enough to act logically."

Several weeks later, he is placed in a board-and-care home and assigned to a case manager who also functions as his payee. He continues in weekly individual therapy with Dr. Dickens.

Homelessness is a widespread societal problem that affects significant numbers of chronically mentally ill individuals; among the homeless, approximately 35% to 40% are chronically mentally ill. The high prevalence of homelessness among these people stems not only from the lack of comprehensive community care systems in many areas, but also, as Mr. Drummond's case illustrates, from the difficulties that severely psychotic individuals have in maintaining themselves in community-based housing.

Thus, merely providing housing for a homeless mentally ill patient is not a solution; in order to be able to maintain a stable residence, the patient must also be successfully engaged in treatment. Engagement, as well as assessment and treatment, of the homeless mentally ill patient is essentially as described in previous chapters regarding chronically mentally ill patients in general.

Engagement and Assessment of the Patient

As in the case of Mr. Drummond, the treatment process begins with engaging the patient in a relationship and performing a comprehensive individualized assessment. This initial step may be the most difficult. Because the appearance of many homeless mentally ill individuals is bizarre and repulsive, residents may easily forget that underneath the repugnant exterior is a scared, vulnerable, and desperate human being, longing for a safe way to make human contact. Residents who succeed in overcoming their initial repugnance can have enormous impacts on the lives of these individuals, and many seemingly untreatable homeless patients, like Mr. Drummond, can have surprisingly successful outcomes.

Engagement and Assessment of the Family

A common misconception about homeless mentally ill persons is that they have no families, so contact with families is often overlooked in the assessment process. Yet, many homeless patients have interested families who can provide, at the least, history that the patient is either unable or unwilling to give, and who may reveal useful information about the patient's past, present, and future functioning and motivation. In addition, the family can reveal the extent to which they wish to remain involved with the patient, as well as their capacity to provide financial or emotional support.

Joseph Drummond (continued from p. 165)

When Dr. Dickens asks Mr. Drummond about his family, he is surprised to find that his father lives in a nearby suburb and that Mr. Drummond speaks to him regularly. Contact with the father reveals him to be a caring and concerned man who has been desperately worried about his son, but has felt helpless to change his son's downward course. The father has continued to supply his son with food and money on occasion, and has even attempted to have him hospitalized. Mr. Drummond, when he was in his paranoid state, felt that his father was trying to kill him; as his condition has cleared up, he now is relieved that his father still cares and can provide emotional and (limited) financial support.

Involving the Treatment System

Most homeless mentally ill individuals require systems supports in order to maintain stable community living. Common supports include case management, payeeship, and supported housing, as well as medication, individual therapy, group treatment, day treatment, and rehabilitative programs. In some cases, like that of Mr. Drummond, services are available and acceptable to the patient, and treatment proceeds smoothly:

Joseph Drummond (continued from above)

Once in the hospital, Mr. Drummond accepts medication, and his psychosis clears considerably. Dr. Dickens arranges for a case manager to assist the patient in coordinating needed services, maintaining his SSI as a source of income, and arranging housing. Because of Mr. Drummond's history of spending his money unwisely, Dr. Dickens recommends that the case manager should initially be made the patient's payee. Even though Mr. Drummond mildly protests this arrangement, he is clearly relieved, for he fears losing his stability and returning to the street. Finally, because of Mr. Drummond's poor performance in his own apartment, Dr. Dickens recommends placement in a board-and-care home, where food and shelter are assured and medications are dispensed, and where there are few intense interactions that might stir up Mr. Drummond's paranoia. Once in this placement, Mr. Drummond is able to maintain a stable residence while continuing to receive medication management and individual therapy from Dr. Dickens.

Prolonged Periods of Hospitalization

Some patients who have been homeless need prolonged periods of hospitalization, often involuntary, as the following case illustrates:

Mr. Markson, a 28-year-old man with a diagnosis of paranoid schizophrenia, had just been hospitalized for the 12th time since the age of 19. On a number of occasions, early in the course of his illness, he had threatened to kill his parents when acutely psychotic, and three times was asked to leave home. On each occasion, he was hospitalized, and his parents, after conferring with his doctor and social worker in the hospital, took him back when he was discharged. Finally, at age 23, he broke his father's wrist and was hospitalized again. This time the parents refused to take him back.

He was placed in a board-and-care home, but was asked to leave after a month because of repeated threats of physical violence. Since then, for 5 years, he has been homeless, sometimes living in shelters, but mostly staying on the streets and in parks. He has wandered from city to city and place to place, only occasionally receiving his SSI check because of his constantly changing whereabouts. He has been totally resistant to taking antipsychotic medications when not in hospitals and has been medicated only with great difficulty during his brief hospitalizations. He has refused all housing placements and referrals to day or outpatient treatment.

On the streets, he is paranoid, guarded, and irritable to the point at which almost any contact with people quickly escalates to physical violence. "Voices" constantly tell him that people want to hurt him. He has had several arrests for assaults on strangers whom he had incorporated into his delusional system; each time he was sent to a psychiatric hospital. During his brief involuntary hospitalizations, he accepted medication and became less paranoid and threatening, but then talked his way out of the hospital and back onto the streets, where the cycle of decompensation began again.

To break the cycle of homelessness and revolving-door hospital admissions, Mr. Markson requires prolonged involuntary hospitalization. His history of persistent psychosis, treatment noncompliance, rapid decompensation, and repeated assaultiveness provides adequate evidence (in most states) for commitment. Yet residents may find it difficult to take this step. State hospital staff may pressure the resident to discharge the patient quickly to keep the census down, or may react angrily to the patient's noncompliance by wanting to put him back in the street.

Residents may also find it hard to initiate commitment with a patient who appears somewhat compensated in the hospital and is insisting he or she wants to leave. In this instance, the patient's history of assaults and noncompliance appears to have more weight in the argument for dangerousness than does his or her immediate mental status, and many judges would be inclined to agree.

In Mr. Markson's case, the inpatient resident was successful in having him committed for 6 months, during which he began to engage in treatment for the first time. He agreed to stay in the hospital voluntarily after the first 6 months, and over the course of the next year was transitioned to a halfway house and day program.

In other cases, such as the following two patients, prolonged and persistent "systems advocacy" by the resident may be required to obtain needed services for the patient and to establish a structure that increases the patient's likelihood of complying with treatment:

Mr. Thomas

Mr. Thomas, a 28-year-old man with a 10-year history of chronic paranoid schizophrenia and polysubstance dependence, is an inpatient in a community psychiatric hospital who is ready for discharge and has nowhere to go. His history of spending his SSI checks almost exclusively on drugs and so running short on rent money has led to numerous evictions from apartments and single-room occupancy hotels, and his frequent aggressive and disruptive behavior in shelters around the city has resulted in his being barred from using them. Community residences will not take him because of his persistent use of drugs and his associated violent behavior. No inpatient drug rehabilitation unit in the city would accept him for treatment because of his dual diagnosis, and a drug treatment program for the dually diagnosed on the other side of the state has a 3-month waiting list. Because his psychotic symptoms are in near remission, the state hospital would not accept him. Even if discharge to private housing would have been appropriate for Mr. Thomas, he has no money up front for rent, and no supplemental funds are available. He has no friends or family.

After multiple phone calls by the social worker and psychiatric resident, a shelter (with a nearby soup kitchen) is found that is willing to give Mr. Thomas another chance. A local outreach team, noted for its work with homeless persons, is contacted; they meet with Mr. Thomas and agree to follow up with him to do what is possible to ensure his compliance with his appointments, injections of medication, and abstinence. The idea of managing Mr. Thomas's limited income for him so he will not use up his monthly check is suggested to him, but he repeatedly refuses.

Despite all this effort, Mr. Thomas is readmitted 1 month after discharge, having used his check on drugs and complaining of suicidal ideation. The resident who had treated him remembers the previous situation and insists that, as a condition of admission to the university hospital, Mr. Thomas sign a contract to turn over his monthly check to a payee. Mr. Thomas reluctantly agrees, because he does not want to remain on the street or go to the state hospital. The resident promptly notifies SSI that Mr. Thomas requires a payee, and a member of the local outreach team is appointed. With this in place, Mr. Thomas is more readily readmitted to his previous shelter and is able to remain there for several months.

The resident realizes that the shelter staff will be able to accept more difficult clients if they feel that they have more psychiatric support. He therefore volunteers to work in the shelter two evenings a week, where he can continue ongoing therapy and medication management with Mr. Thomas.

After a few months in the shelter, Mr. Thomas expresses interest in a more stable residence, but no mental health residence will take him because of his substance addiction. At first he is discouraged, but his resident and the staff at the shelter place him on the waiting list at the state dual-diagnosis program. They point out that he can stay at the shelter 3 more months until he gets in that program. With the support of his resident therapist and the shelter staff, Mr. Thomas ultimately succeeds in maintaining sobriety and being placed in a long-term residence.

Ms. Harrison

Ms. Harrison, 48 years of age, is well known to all the psychiatric emergency rooms and hospitals in the area because of her long history of severe psychosis, homelessness, multiple medical problems, and noncompliant and disruptive behavior. She has accumulated a tally of at least 15 admissions to the local state hospital and more than 50 admissions to local acute care psychiatric units.

She presents to the university psychiatric emergency room at 3:00 A.M., requesting admission because she has "nowhere to go." She is carrying a paper bag full of clothes and 10 bottles of medicine, which was prescribed for her at the state hospital 14 days ago. She does not know what her medications are for or how to take them.

After the interview, a physical examination shows early signs of congestive heart failure, although not severe enough to warrant admission to a medical unit. The resident is sure, however, that if she continues to wander the street and does not take her medications, her heart condition will become worse. Shelters throughout the city are called, but all of the shelters refuse her, saying her behavior has been consistently disruptive and unmanageable. Her catchment area emergency room, where she had presented earlier in the evening, is then called with concerns about the decline in her medical and psychiatric conditions, but the clinician there says that she is not sick enough to warrant admission and that there is nothing that can be done because "she never follows through with treatment." Because of her obvious inability to care for herself, her deteriorating physical condition, and the lack of any alternative disposition, Ms. Harrison is admitted to the university psychiatric service, but is once again transferred to the state hospital because of no alternative disposition plans.

At this point the resident decides to call the state hospital physician who is caring for Ms. Harrison, reporting that he has some information on her that might be helpful. The state hospital physician is receptive, stating that he does not want to discharge Ms. Harrison to the streets, but that he has no information on which to base a commitment petition. The resident's information about her inability to care for herself and her deteriorating condition is exactly what the state hospital needs to obtain a commitment.

In the health system, flow of accurate information can never be taken for granted; many apparent system failures that lead to homelessness are due to inadequate communication of key data.

Long-Term Outcome

As homeless mentally ill persons grow older, some of them may ultimately find life on the streets intolerable and so can be ready for a change in life-style. Engagement in treatment may become possible at this point, either in an inpatient or outpatient setting, and significant improvement may result, as in the following case:

Mr. James, a 32-year-old, single man, was first hospitalized at age 18 with a diagnosis of schizophrenia, paranoid type. He left his home in the midwest in his early 20s and has wandered about the country since, with psychiatric hospitalizations at least once a year. He has never worked, nor has he been on SSI. His income has come from selling drugs, panhandling, and armed robbery; he has had one arrest for grand theft and several arrests for armed robbery.

For the most part, he has lived on the streets for the past 8 years, occasionally staying in a motel, and domiciled in hospitals and jails for relatively brief periods. No attempt has ever been made to commit him to long-term involuntary hospitalization. He has been delusional and hallucinating almost continuously for 8 years, but has refused to take neuroleptic medications except when in hospitals. At least once a week he becomes intoxicated on alcohol or drugs to drown out the "voices."

In the 3 months before his current hospital admission, he became increasingly disorganized, depressed, and tormented by the voices telling him to kill himself and others. After he was viciously assaulted and robbed of his few belongings and left unconscious, he was brought to the hospital.

Now, with his psychosis stabilized, he tells his assigned resident that he fears that he cannot survive on the streets any longer and that for the first time he really wants to get some help. The resident begins to form a treatment relationship with Mr. James and arranges to contact his family. SSI is applied for, and the patient is eventually placed in a board-and-care home. A year later, he is still living in the board-and-care home and seeing the resident for medication and therapy.

Rehabilitation

While placement in stable housing is an important objective for the homeless mentally ill patient, it is not the final endpoint of treatment. In fact, placement in stable housing is often the vehicle that permits further rehabilitation to occur. Thus, a patient may engage in treatment, stabilize sufficiently to obtain and maintain housing, and then proceed to attain further rehabilitative goals.

Joseph Drummond (continued from p. 167)

Once Mr. Drummond is placed in a board-and-care home, he continues to progress in his treatment with Dr. Dickens. As his mental status improves, he is able to formulate more appropriate goals and work toward them. His hygiene and appearance improve, and he now passes in the streets unnoticed. He begins a day treatment program, obtains a part-time job, saves his money, and gets his own apartment.

By the time Dr. Dickens completes his residency, Mr. Drummond's paranoia is markedly reduced. The patient works full time in the university library, has his own apartment, and is taking a course at night. He continues to abuse alcohol and marijuana on occasion, but is beginning, in therapy, to consider becoming abstinent. He has regular visits with his father and feels good about himself and his life.

Mr. Drummond, reflecting on the 3 years of treatment, comments to Dr. Dickens: "You know, when I first met you, I thought I was beyond hope. But you seemed like you really cared. So I thought, 'What have I got to lose?' But I never realized I could have so much to gain."

Conclusions

The chronically mentally ill patient presents the clinician with formidable challenges at every stage of treatment. Because, however, many of these challenges can yield to skillful, persistent effort, the care of this patient population can be very rewarding to psychiatric clinicians. Yet, because these patients are so severely impaired, clinicians who work with them must learn a broad range of treatment strategies and interventions.

In this guide we have discussed and illustrated a variety of approaches to the care of chronically mentally ill patients, together with the clinical contexts in which these approaches are likely to prove useful. We trust that the guide has helped you understand how each segment of treatment works, how the treatment interventions come together, and how a coherent treatment strategy can be formulated when you are faced with a patient whose situation is complex and confusing.

Because the rehabilitation and recovery of patients with chronic mental illness often span decades, as a resident you can participate in only a limited segment of each patient's clinical course. It is not easy, therefore, for you to see the long-range results of the cumulative efforts of the many clinicians involved in a patient's care. We hope, however, that the relatively limited exposure during your residency to these individuals, among the most impaired of our patients, will encourage you later on to seek out opportunities to help them to overcome their disabilities, to become useful and contributing members of society, and to lead lives that preserve their dignity and self-respect.

Appendix A

Biopsychosocial Assessment Protocol

This protocol for the biopsychosocial assessment of patients with chronic mental illness is based on an individualized, longitudinal, multidimensional life-course perspective that goes beyond diagnosis to address adaptation to and rehabilitation of the illness (see pp. 38 and 71).

I. Longitudinal perspective

A. Chronological assessment

Each of the following systems is assessed longitudinally and chronologically. Data from each system can be organized on a time line so that the causal and temporal relationships between significant events in different systems can be readily identified.

B. Assessment of baseline

In each system, periods of medication compliance and noncompliance must be clearly identified. Accurate assessment of functioning in any system depends on knowing whether the patient is at baseline or is decompensating.

C. Assessment of life course

The following life-course questions are applicable to each of the four interacting systems discussed below:

This protocol is substantially based on a presentation by K. Minkoff and R. Stern at the 31st annual meeting of the Institute of Hospital & Community Psychiatry, Boston, Massachusetts, 1980.

- Are there observable patterns that seem to repeat over time?
- How adaptive are these patterns?
- Do they contribute to growth or stability, or to regression?
- Do the patterns change or remain the same?
- What factors contribute to growth or stability, or to regression?
- In what direction is the patient's career moving?

II. Multidimensional assessment

A. Assessment of the illness

Assessing the illness includes evaluating the range of symptoms of disordered thinking, feeling, and behavior, and the response of these symptoms to treatment.

Symptoms:

- What are the specific thinking, feeling, and behavioral symptoms?
- How severe and persistent are they?
- Are there times when the patient is asymptomatic?

Response to medication:

- Do symptoms respond to medication? In what way?
- Do some symptoms respond more than others?
- Has the patient received an adequate medication trial at an appropriate dosage?
- What has been the history of medication compliance?
- How are symptoms related to periods of compliance?

Side effects:

- Does the patient have akathisia, akinesia, tremor, tardive dyskinesia, or other troublesome side effects from medication?

Additional medical and psychiatric illness:

- Does the patient also suffer from substance abuse or dependence, mental retardation, seizure disorder, neurological disorders, metabolic or endocrine disorder, etc.?

B. Assessment of the individual

Assessing the individual includes evaluating the varied intrapsychic, developmental, and stylistic factors that characterize the individual's adaptation to illness.

Premorbid functioning:

- What was the patient like before the onset of illness?

- What were his or her strengths, goals, and typical personality patterns?
- What were his or her developmental issues at the time of the onset of illness?
- What meaning did the onset of illness have to him or her?

Adaptational pattern to illness: Patients demonstrate a range of adaptational patterns that change over time.

- Is the patient frightened by illness?
- Has the patient found a method of self-soothing?
- Does the patient deny the illness, as opposed to being realistically aware of the deficits and difficulties?
- How accepting is the patient of the prolonged nature of the illness?
- How much has coping with the illness become integrated successfully into the patient's life?
- How does the patient cope with shame, guilt, stigma, despair, and narcissistic injury associated with the illness?
- How did the onset of illness change the patient's life?
- How does the patient accept his or her need for medication and ongoing treatment?
- How institutionalized and compliant or stridently independent and noncompliant is the patient?
- Can the patient ask for help when needed?
- What is the patient's baseline when medication compliant and sober, and how has that baseline changed over time?

Existential concerns:

- What is the meaning to the individual of having chronic mental illness?
- What makes life worth living for the patient?
- Are there friends, family, jobs, hobbies, or special interests that are sustaining?
- Does the patient have a realistic life plan given his or her illness?
- Are there attainable goals?

Strengths:

- What have been the social, vocational, and educational skills of the patient before and after the onset of illness?
- What are the patient's abilities to manage activities of daily living such as self-care, cooking, traveling, and living alone?

Patterns of growth and maturation:

- How has the patient handled normative developmental stages such as leaving home, career choice, sexual identity, and choice of mate?

- Which have been successfully resolved, and which are still sources of conflict or struggle?
- Where has the patient given up?
- What is the next desired maturational step?

Character style:

- What personality style dominates the clinical picture?
- Is the person predominantly paranoid, schizoid, antisocial, histrionic, phobic, dependent, or impulsive?

Primary and secondary gain:

- What are the intrapsychic and environmental gratifications derived by the patient from illness?
- How many of these lead to resistance to change and manipulation of the therapeutic or other relationships?

C. **Assessment of the family**

Assessing the family includes evaluating the adaptational patterns of the family unit over the course of the patient's illness.

Information about the illness:

- How much does the family know about the patient's mental illness, its treatment, and its course?
- How willing and able are they to make use of that knowledge to understand and help the patient?

Familial adaptational patterns: Understanding the history, growth, and development of the family, and the typical patterns of crisis management, is crucial.

- Are problems with the patient handled with the same ease or difficulty as other family problems?
- Before the onset of illness, how did the family function?

Family adaptation to the illness:

- How did the onset of illness affect each family member?
- How did the family respond as a system?
- What is the level of denial?
- How does the family support medication compliance and treatment compliance?
- What system has the family evolved for providing support to the patient, and, conversely, for setting limits on the patient?

- How are stress and conflict resolved?
- How are decisions made?
- What is the family's position about the patient's living at home?
- How does the family experience the loss of the patient as a functioning member?
- What hopes have been disappointed? What hopes remain?
- Does the family have attainable goals for the patient?

Relationship of the family atmosphere to the patient's symptoms and function:

- What effects does the family have on the patient's morbidity or role performance, as evaluated through congruence of the patient's and the family's expectations for behavior and performance?
- What is the level of stress or stimulation in the family?
- How do family stresses affect the patient's level of stability or progress?

Degree of separation/individuation:

- To what extent has the patient become emotionally independent of family conflicts?
- How do other family disturbances affect the patient's course?

Burden on the family:

- To what degree is the patient's illness a burden for the family?
- Can the family rely on outside supports to ameliorate the burden?
- When the patient is symptomatic, does he or she risk total rejection?
- What is the family's financial status?

Impending losses:

- Are there potential changes in the family that could have a subsequent impact on the patient's course?

Family culture:

- Are there ethnic or cultural variations that affect the way mental illness is perceived and the way "abnormal" symptoms or behaviors are defined?
- How do these attitudes affect treatment relationships?

D. **Assessment of the community and the community care system**

Assessing the community includes evaluating the degree to which the patient's treatment system and larger community can assist or impede progress.

Community support system: For the majority of chronically mentally ill patients, the treatment system is the major community support.

- Is it an adequate system providing a range of program options, including case management, vocational rehabilitation, day treatment and social rehabilitation, community residences, outpatient medication management and psychotherapy, crisis intervention, public and private hospitalization, and substance abuse and dual-diagnosis programs?
- How easily can a patient become involved in these alternatives?
- Are residents part of the decision-making process so that they can facilitate a coordinated program?
- How comprehensive, continuous, and resilient are the programs?
- Does the system assume full case management responsibility?
- What are the "cracks" in the system?
- Are there accessible self-help programs for patients and families?

Patient's treatment system:

- What has been the course of the patient's treatment?
- Have there been significant successes and failures? Has medication compliance been maintained?
- Have the patient and family made significant therapeutic attachments? Have these been helpful?
- What has been the impact of disruptions or losses in therapist or other treatment relationships?
- What behaviors or disabilities have led to treatment failures?
- Does the patient have realistic plans and goals within the treatment system?
- What treatment leverage is available?
- Who are the patient's case managers, and what level of responsibility do they assume?
- What are the patient's programmatic needs?
- Are appropriate resources available?
- Is the patient or family motivated to accept these resources if offered?

Patient's legal status:

- What is the patient's legal status?
- Is treatment voluntary or involuntary?
- Is the patient committable?
- Is medication compliance voluntary or coerced?
- Is medication guardianship advisable, and would the family support it?

- Is the patient competent to manage funds, or is a conservatorship or payeeship advisable?
- Is the patient on probation or parole?
- Is treatment a condition of probation, and if so, how would it be enforced?

Economic and residential support:

- Does the patient have enough income for survival in the local community?
- Are there additional sources of income, as from family, workshop, SSI, SSDI, or Aid for Dependent Children?
- Does the patient have adequate housing?
- Do the living arrangements meet the patient's needs?

The home community:

- Where does the home community stand with respect to political, economic, and social acceptance of mentally ill persons?
- Does the community provide affordable, stable, and adequate housing, transportation, social services, medical care, jobs, inexpensive restaurants, and recreational programs?

Appendix B

Hospital System Assessment Protocol

The structure and function of the treatment unit

1. What is the mission of the unit?
2. What types of patients does the unit prefer to treat?
3. What types of patients does the unit prefer *not* to treat?
4. What are the requirements for admission (clinical, financial, prescreening, etc.)?
5. What are the expectations or requirements for patient behavior and medication compliance, and how are they enforced?
6. What privileges exist, and how are they earned?
7. What sanctions or restrictions exist, and how are they applied?
8. What are the minimum, maximum, and modal expected lengths of stay?
9. What are the fiscal and utilization review determinants of length of stay?
10. What are the clinical determinants of length of stay?
11. What are the criteria for readmission?

This protocol is discussed briefly on p. 62.

12. What resources are available to back up the unit in the event of the following?:

    a. Violence
    b. Suicidal behavior
    c. Placement difficulties
    d. Need for state hospital transfer
    e. Short or long-term involuntary commitment
    f. Homeless patients requiring administrative discharge or leaving AMA
    g. Need for emergency case management or aftercare

13. What are the guidelines for the following?:

    a. Transfer to a more secure setting
    b. Seclusion and restraint
    c. AMA and administrative discharge
    d. Dealing with homeless patients
    e. Referral for aftercare

Unit authority and responsibility

1. How is the organization chart set up?

2. Who is administratively in charge?

3. Who is clinically in charge, and how do clinical decisions get made?

4. Who are the therapist and case manager for each patient?

5. How are administrative and clinical disputes resolved? What happens when clinical considerations are opposed to administrative considerations?

6. What is the resident's role, and how much authority does he or she have?

7. Who backs up or validates the resident's decisions before they are implemented? (The team? The head nurse? The service chief?)

Appendix C

Community System Assessment Protocol

For each program within each category, obtain and record the following data:

- *Name* of program
- *Address* and *phone number*
- *Names of director* and *key contact person(s)* for referrals
- *Purpose* of the program
- *Eligibility criteria:* clinical, demographic, financial
- *Disability level* of appropriate clients
- *Requirements for participation:* attendance, financial, medication compliance, participation in additional treatment, etc.
- *Discharge criteria:* criteria for successful completion of the program, and behaviors that will result in administrative discharge

Categories of System Resources

Within each category are listed specific questions to be used for defining the range and scope of services within that category for a particular care system.

A. Case management

1. How is case management defined in the system? Does it include the following?:
    - Brokering of treatment resources

This protocol is discussed briefly on pp. 65 and 136.

- Developing system-wide treatment plans
- Directing treatment decisions by directing and coordinating treatment providers
- Providing "management" services, such as budgeting, payeeship for SSI, etc.
- Providing treatment services, such as counseling, day treatment, residential programming, and vocational rehabilitation

2. Is there a defined case management program in the area, or is case management provided within each program, or both? If there is a distinct case management program, which of the above case management services are provided by the program?
3. What are the eligibility criteria to receive case management?
4. Are case managers empowered to manage clients' funds?
5. Are case managers empowered to mandate treatment assignments, or only to make referrals?
6. What is the average case management caseload?
7. What is the clinician's own role in providing case management, as defined by the system, by the program in which he or she works, and by himself or herself? Does the clinician decide what services the case manager arranges?

B. Income support

1. What income support programs are available to mentally ill individuals in this area? Do they include the following?:
    - Supplemental Security Income (SSI)
    - Social Security Disability Insurance (SSDI)
    - General relief or welfare
    - Veterans' benefits
    - Food stamps
2. What are the eligibility criteria and application processes for each benefit?
3. How much money is available from each source?
4. Are housing supports available and by what mechanism?
5. What health care benefits, such as Medicaid and Medicare, are available in association with income supports?
6. What types of psychiatric care are covered?
7. What are the criteria for determining the need for a payeeship for SSI or SSDI if the patient cannot manage his or her own funds?

8. How are such payeeships established and administered?

C. Outpatient treatment

1. What outpatient programs are available, and what are the clinical, financial, and residential eligibility requirements for each?
2. What is the intake and referral process? Is there a waiting list for intake? For therapist assignment? For psychiatric evaluation?
3. Does the program provide individual case management as well as therapy?
4. Are families involved? Individually or in psychoeducational groups? Short-term or long-term?
5. What therapeutic modalities are provided? Are there groups for chronically mentally ill patients?
6. What is the relationship between the psychiatrist and other clinical specialists? How is medication provided, and how closely is compliance monitored?
7. What provisions are made for continuity of care between the outpatient program and other system components?

D. Inpatient treatment

1. What are the available private general hospital psychiatric units within the system?
2. For each hospital, what are the clinical, demographic, and financial criteria for admission? Does the hospital accept voluntary or involuntary patients? adolescents or elderly? Does the hospital accept Medicaid, Medicare, or self-pay? What is the admission process?
3. For the state or other public hospital, what are the admission criteria, and what is the admission process? Is there a defined prescreening program?
4. Does the state hospital accept long-term patients who are so sick that they fall through the cracks elsewhere in the system, or does it function more as a short-term revolving-door setting? Do all patients have to be committable?
5. What are the levels of disability tolerated at different hospitals? Is participation in groups mandatory? Is the milieu intense, or is it low-key?
6. Does the hospital accept dual-diagnosis patients, medically ill patients, or mentally retarded patients?

7. For each hospital, who are the "gatekeepers"?
8. How quickly can admission be arranged? Can the resident authorize admission, or only request admission? How likely is the resident's request to be denied?
9. Are there alternatives to hospitalization, such as crisis residences or respite programs, and if so, how are they accessed?

E. Emergency services

1. What is the 24-hour emergency capacity in the system? How do patients gain access to it? Is it located in a particular site or sites, or is it mobile? How much outreach and follow-up are provided?

F. Day treatment/social rehabilitation

1. What types of day treatment and social rehabilitation programs are available in the area? Do they include the following?:
   a. Partial hospitalization (as an alternative to acute inpatient treatment)
   b. Day treatment (long term, goal oriented, rehabilitation focused)
   c. Day activity (long term, maintenance oriented—for lower functioning clients)
   d. Clubhouse model social rehabilitation (i.e., Fountain House model, a membership-oriented program that is based on the assumption that rehabilitation derives from participation in clubhouse functions)
   e. Social clubs and drop-in centers (i.e., loosely structured social support and recreation)
2. For each program, what are the eligibility criteria, referral process, length of stay, and participation requirements?
3. What level of patient functioning is appropriate?
4. Is there a waiting list, and if so, how is it prioritized?
5. What happens to clients who do not make progress at the expected rate?
6. Does the program provide individualized case management, family education, or family therapy?
7. How does the program link up with other parts of the care system?

8. What are the policies regarding substance abuse, medication compliance, attendance, and relapse? How are "violations" dealt with?
9. What happens to clients who graduate or terminate? Is there an alumni or aftercare program? Is there a less intensive "step down" program?

G. Residential programs

1. What types of residential programs are available in the area? Do they include the following?:

   - *Short-term crisis residences:* for respite from existing living situations, or as an alternative to acute hospitalization.
   - *Dormitory or inn programs:* low-expectation settings (usually on state hospital grounds) with slightly less supervision than acute-care settings.
   - *Quarterway houses:* low-expectation settings, usually at or near a hospital, but with a group-home format.
   - *Halfway house/community residences:* medium- to high-expectation settings, with a group-home format and 24-hour staff. They may or may not be transitional.
   - *Cooperative apartments:* higher-expectation settings, usually transitional to independent living and usually with less than 24-hour staffing.
   - *Foster care:* individual placements in private homes with variable levels of support.
   - *Board-and-care homes:* low-expectation rooming-house model with meals and varying levels of supervision and programming.
   - *Nursing homes:* generic nursing care facilities, with varying levels of nursing care and varying accessibility to chronically mentally ill patients.
   - *Intermediate care facilities:* low-expectation settings, intermediate-level chronic care facilities specifically geared to mentally ill residents.
   - *Supervised independent living:* individual or group living settings with intermittent staff support.
   - *Shelters:* transitional residences for homeless individuals.
   - *Patient-specific residences:* for dual-diagnosis patients with and without mandated abstinence; for adolescent, elderly, mentally ill, and retarded persons, etc.

2. For each program, what are the eligibility criteria, referral processes, and expected length of stay?

3. What are the financial requirements and reimbursement mechanisms?
4. What level of functioning is appropriate for a referred patient?
5. Is there a waiting list, and if so, how is it prioritized, and how are admission decisions made?
6. What are the requirements for participation? Are clients expected to attend a day program, perform chores, be medication compliant, or remain abstinent? What sanctions are imposed for failure to comply with program rules?
7. What level of staffing coverage is available?
8. Are meals or housekeeping provided, or do residents cook and/or clean for themselves?
9. Do residents have their own rooms, or do they share rooms?
10. Does the program have a group-home milieu format or an individualized format?
11. Does the program provide individual case management and/or financial supervision? If so, to what extent?
12. What is the linkage of the program to other components of the care system?
13. Are there limits on hospitalization in order to remain in the program?
14. How much mobility and spending money and how many other freedoms are residents allowed?
15. Are there specific programs for the homeless? Are they separate, or are they affiliated with shelters? What services do these programs provide?

H. Vocational rehabilitation programs

1. What types of vocational rehabilitation programs are available in the area? Do they include the following?:
   - Vocational training and education
   - Prevocational clubhouse or day treatment
   - Work programs
   - Sheltered workshops
   - Transitional employment (i.e., temporary placements in competitive jobs)
   - Supported competitive employment (i.e., placement in jobs with support)
   - Job placement services

2. Do mental health agencies, state vocational rehabilitation agencies, or private rehabilitation agencies sponsor the various programs?
3. What are the eligibility criteria, referral processes, and expected length of placement for each program type?
4. What level of disability is best served by each program?
5. Are placements intended to be temporary or long-term?
6. What level of expectation—in terms of attendance, productivity, and behavior—is associated with each program type? What consequences occur when clients fail to meet program expectations?
7. What levels of individual case management and group support are provided?

I. Self-help programs

1. What self-help programs are available for mentally ill individuals in this area? Do they include Recovery, Inc.; Schizophrenics Anonymous; or affective disorder support groups?
2. What self-help programs such as the Alliance for the Mentally Ill are available for families of the mentally ill?
3. What are the eligibility criteria for each program?
4. What types of patients or families are best suited for each program?
5. Are meetings support oriented, education oriented, or both?
6. Are professionals welcome to attend?
7. Are meeting schedules and literature available?
8. How are referrals best made?

J. Treatment resources for substance abuse

1. What substance abuse programs are available in the area? Do they include the following?:
   - Detoxification
   - Inpatient rehabilitation
   - Day treatment rehabilitation
   - Sober houses
   - Halfway houses (short-term)
   - Outpatient counseling
   - Dual-diagnosis programs (inpatient, outpatient, or residential)

- Self-help (12-step programs such as AA, NA, CA, etc.)
- Dual-diagnosis groups—"double trouble"

2. What are the eligibility criteria, referral processes, length of stay, and requirements for participation in each program?
3. To what extent are patients with dual diagnosis acceptable? Which medications are permissible?
4. What level of functioning is necessary for a patient to participate effectively?
5. Is abstinence mandatory at the outset, or is it a goal to be achieved?
6. Is the program operated primarily within the addiction system or the mental health system?
7. For self-help programs, are meeting schedules available? Which meetings are best suited for dual-diagnosis patients? Which meetings are professionals welcome to attend?

K. Generic medical and social services

1. Where do mentally ill individuals obtain general medical care? What types of services are available?
2. For homebound, infirm, or physically ill clients, are visiting nurse, meals-on-wheels, or homemaking services available?
3. What types of day care are available for clients with children?
4. What types of public transportation and transportation assistance are available?
5. Do patients have access to public libraries, YMCA, swimming pools, etc?

Appendix D

The Legal System: A Guide to Basic Knowledge

A. Commitment

- What are the specific legal criteria for commitment, both emergency and long-term? What is the process for initiating commitment?
- What is the duration of emergency and long-term commitment? What is the process for judicial review?
- If a person is committable, what steps are necessary to contain and transport him or her to a secure unit?
- Under what circumstances can commitment proceedings be instituted by families? police officers? nonphysicians?
- How much discretion does the law give to the physician in various clinical situations? For example, how immediate must the risk be to self or others? How severe must a person's inability to care for himself or herself be?
- What are the laws governing criminal commitment for pretrial evaluation following arrest? for aid in sentencing? for ongoing treatment?
- Is there legal provision for outpatient commitment? If so, how does it work?

B. Involuntary treatment

- What are the legal criteria for emergency and ongoing involuntary

---

This guide is referred to on p. 69.

treatment, specifically with medication?

- What legal process must be followed to administer involuntary medication? Does it require judicial review, or only administrative review? Does the patient have to be declared incompetent? Is the appointment of a legal guardian required?
- Can families or physicians be legally empowered to enforce medication compliance when patients are no longer in the hospital?
- Does the decision to administer involuntary medication depend on "substituted judgment" (i.e., what the patient would do if he or she were capable of deciding), or only on the physician's determination of the patient's best interest?
- What sanctions can be applied to patients on parole or probation who refuse recommended follow-up? Can the threat of jail be realistically implemented? For which types of patients?

C. Competency

- What are the legal criteria for declaring a patient incompetent to make treatment decisions, to manage money, or to stand trial?
- What is the process of competency determination in each of these areas?
- What happens when a patient is declared incompetent? Is a conservator, guardian, or payee appointed? How is the guardian or other protector chosen?

Appendix E

Sample Behavior Contract

The purpose of this type of contract, referred to on p. 132, is to clarify expectations for the patient's performance of specific chores or rehabilitative tasks, in return for defined rewards.

We agree to give B. $25 per week out of his SSI check for basic spending money. In addition, $25 per week will be set aside for board, and $35 per month will be used to pay bills and necessities. (Beginning June 1, unauthorized charges will be deducted from spending money.) The remaining $25 per week will be available *to be earned* by B. according to the attached weekly checklist form [see p. 196].

B. will earn one point for each task done each day (including one point for each hour of yard work), and one point for each half day of work or day treatment.

Scoring will take place *daily*, after dinner, on the weekly checklist. If *no tasks* are done in an entire day, the score will be –2. If, at any time during the day, B. refuses to cooperate when asked to help with a family project, he will lose two points. The weekly total of points will be given to B. (or deducted, if the total is negative) in dollars as *additional* spending money (over and above the basic $25).

The scoring system may be revised in the future as needed.

Money not earned will be saved for B.'s future needs, as determined by his father.

_________________________	_________________________
Signed/Dated **Patient**	Signed/Dated **Parent(s)**

____

Witnessed
Clinician

B.'s Weekly Checklist

B. earns one point for each task done each day (including one point for each hour of yard work), and one point for each half day of work or day treatment.

If no tasks are done the entire day, the score shall be −2 for the day. If B. refuses to cooperate on a family project during the day, two points will be subtracted from the weekly total.

Weekly total _______

Total for the week _______

Appendix F

Alcohol and Drug Intake Assessment

1. Tell me about your drinking/drugging pattern. What do you drink? Do you drink/drug every day? How many drinks? How much alcohol do you put in each drink? Do you measure the alcohol?
2. How much alcohol do you consume in a week?
3. Was there ever a time in your life when you worried about your alcohol or drug intake? Have you ever tried to control the amount/frequency?
4. Have you ever taken any drugs? [Mention pot, cocaine, speed, acid, PCP, tranquilizers.] Has a doctor ever prescribed tranquilizers for you? [Get name and dosage.]
5. Does anyone in your family have a problem with drinking or taking drugs?
6. Is anyone in your family concerned about your drinking?
7. What do you do to relax or unwind, or calm down? What do you do if you cannot get to sleep at night?
8. Have you ever taken a drink/drug in the morning?
9. Do you have any health problems that may relate to alcohol/drugs? [Suggest specific problems.]
10. Are your caregivers concerned about your drinking/drugging?

This protocol is briefly discussed on pp. 151 and 153.

11. Have you gotten in trouble at your treatment program because of alcohol/drugs? Have you been suspended or terminated?
12. Have alcohol and drugs led to emergency room visits? to hospitalizations?
13. Have you ever lost time from work because of drinking or because you were sick from drinking?
14. Have you ever been in a motor vehicle accident or another dangerous situation in which alcohol/drugs were involved? Who was driving? Were alcohol/drugs involved?
15. Have you ever been arrested for driving under the influence (DUI)?
16. Do you know what a blackout is? Have you ever had a blackout when you were drinking? How often?
17. Does it annoy you if someone tells you that you drank too much?
18. Has there been an increase in the amount of drugs/alcohol you used in the last 6 to 12 months?
19. Do you seem to be able to "hold your liquor" better than others you know? Does it take more alcohol or drugs to get you "feeling good" than it does others?
20. Have you ever tried to cut down on the amounts or kinds of alcohol and/or drugs? (See question 3.)
21. Have you ever tried to quit?
22. Have you ever felt guilty after drinking or drugging?
23. Have you ever lied about drinking or the amounts you drank?
24. Have you ever "gotten drunk" even when you had planned not to?
25. If you do drink or use drugs, what do you like about this activity? What, if anything, don't you like?
26. Do you find that drugs and alcohol are helpful or unhelpful in dealing with your mental illness? In what ways?
27. What effect does getting drunk or high have on your symptoms? How about when you are coming down, hung over, or crashing?

After asking these questions, ask yourself [i.e., the interviewer] how you feel. Do you feel the person has been defensive or uncomfortable because of the questions? Does your "gut" feeling tell you there is more to the story than he or she is letting on? If so, then there probably is.

Selected Reading List

General References

Bachrach LL: Deinstitutionalization: An Analytical Review and Sociological Perspective. Rockville, MD, National Institute of Mental Health, 1976

Bachrach LL: Leona Bachrach Speaks: Selected Speeches and Lectures. New Directions for Mental Health Services, No 35, San Francisco, CA, Jossey-Bass, 1987

Bachrach LL, Nadelson CC (eds): Treating Chronically Mentally Ill Women. Washington, DC, American Psychiatric Press, 1988

Bellack AS (ed): Schizophrenia: Treatment, Management and Rehabilitation. Orlando, FL, Grune & Stratton, 1984

Cohen NL (ed): Psychiatry Takes to the Streets: Outreach and Crisis Intervention for the Mentally Ill. New York, Guilford, 1990

Faulkner LR, Cutler DL, Krohn DD, et al: A basic residency curriculum concerning the chronically mentally ill. Am J Psychiatry 146:1323–1327, 1989

Geller JL: Cinical guidelines for the use of involuntary outpatient treatment. Hosp Community Psychiatry 41:749–755, 1990

Goldfinger SM, Hopkin JT, Surber RW: Treatment resisters or system resisters: towards a better service system for acute care recidivists, in Advances in Treating the Young Adult Chronic Patient. New Directions for Mental Health Services No 21. Edited by Pepper B, Ryglewicz H. San Francisco, CA, Jossey-Bass, 1984, pp 17–27

Greenfeld D: The Psychotic Patient: Medication and Psychotherapy. New York, Free Press, 1985

Group for the Advancement of Psychiatry: The Chronic Mental Patient in the Community (GAP Rept No 102). New York, Mental Health Materials Center, 1978

Group for the Advancement of Psychiatry: Interactive Fit: A Guide to Nonpsychotic Chronic Patients (GAP Rept No 121). New York, Brunner/Mazel, 1987

Group for the Advancement of Psychiatry: The Mental Health Professional and the Legal System (GAP Rept No 131). New York, Brunner/Mazel, 1991

Group for the Advancement of Psychiatry: Beyond Symptom Suppression: Improving Long-Term Outcomes of Schizophrenia (GAP Rept No 134). Washington, DC, American Psychiatric Press, 1992

Harding CM, Zubin J, Strauss JS: Chronicity in schizophrenia: fact, partial fact, or artifact? Hosp Community Psychiatry 38:477–486, 1987

Harris M, Bachrach LL (eds): Clinical Case Management. New Directions for Mental Health Services No 40. San Francisco, CA, Jossey-Bass, 1988

Herz MI, Keith SJ, Docherty JP: Psychosocial Treatment of Schizophrenia. Handbook of Schizophrenia, Vol 4 (Nasrallah HA, editor-in-chief). Amsterdam, Elsevier, 1990

Hogarty GE, Anderson CM, Reiss DJ, et al: Family psychoeducation, social skills training, and maintenance chemotherapy in the aftercare treatment of schizophrenia, I: one-year effects of a controlled study on relapse and expressed emotion. Arch Gen Psychiatry 43:633–642, 1986

Kanter JS (ed): Clinical Issues in Treating the Chronically Mentally Ill. New Directions for Mental Health Services No 27. San Francisco, CA, Jossey-Bass, 1985

Lamb HR: Treating the Long-Term Mentally Ill. San Francisco, CA, Jossey-Bass, 1982

Lamb HR: Young adult chronic patients: the new drifters. Hosp Community Psychiatry 33:465–468, 1982

Liberman RP (ed): Psychiatric Rehabilitation of Chronic Mental Patients. Washington, DC, American Psychiatric Press, 1988

McEvoy JP, Freter S, Everett G, et al: Insight and the clinical outcome of schizophrenic patients. J Nerv Ment Dis 177:48–51, 1989

Mendel WM: Treating Schizophrenia. San Francisco, CA, Jossey-Bass, 1989

Menninger WW, Hannah GT (eds): The Chronic Mental Patient II. Washington, DC, American Psychiatric Press, 1987

Meyerson AT (ed): Barriers to Treating the Chronic Mentally Ill. New Directions for Mental Health Services, No 33. San Francisco, CA, Jossey-Bass, 1987

Minkoff K: Beyond deinstitutionalization: a new ideology for the post-institutional era. Hosp Community Psychiatry 38:945–950, 1987a

Minkoff K: Resistance of mental health professionals to working with the chronic mentally ill, in Barriers to Treating the Chronic Mentally Ill. New Directions for Mental Health Services No 33. Edited by Meyerson AT. San Francisco, CA, Jossey-Bass, 1987b, pp 3–20

Minkoff K, Stern R: Paradoxes faced by residents being trained in the psychosocial treatment of people with chronic schizophrenia. Hosp Community Psychiatry 36:859–864, 1985

Nielsen AC III, Stein LI, Talbott JA, et al: Encouraging psychiatrists to work with chronic patients: opportunities and limitations of residency education. Hosp Community Psychiatry 32:767–775, 1981

Pepper B, Kirshner MC, Ryglewicz H: The young adult chronic patient: overview of a population. Hosp Community Psychiatry 32:463–469, 1981

Schwartz SR, Goldfinger SM: The new chronic patient: clinical characteristics of an emerglng subgroup. Hosp Community Psychiatry 32:470–474, 1981

Seeman MV, Greben SE (eds): Office Treatment of Schizophrenia. Washington, DC, American Psychiatric Press, 1990

Stein LI, Test MA, Marx AJ: Alternative to the hospital: a controlled study, Am J Psychiatry 132:517–522, 1975

Strauss JS, Hafez H, Lieberman P, et al: The course of psychiatric disorder, III: longitudinal principles. Am J Psychiatry 142:289–296,1985

Strauss JS, Boker W, Brenner HD (eds): Psychosocial Treatment of Schizophrenia. Toronto, Hans Huber, 1987

Talbott JA: Successful Treatment of the Chronic Mentally Ill: Treatment, Programs, Systems. New York, Human Sciences Press, 1981

Talbott JA (ed): The Chronic Mental Patient: Five Years Later. New York, Grune & Stratton, 1984a

Talbott JA: The patient: first or last? Hosp Community Psychiatry 35:341–344, 1984b

Talbott JA: The Perspective of John Talbott. New Directions for Mental Health Services, No 37. San Francisco, CA, Jossey-Bass, 1988

Self–Reports

Anonymous: "Can we talk?" The schizophrenic patient in psychotherapy. Am J Psychiatry 143:68–70, 1986

Deegan P: Recovery: the lived experience of rehabilitation. Psychosocial Rehabilitation Journal 11:11–19, 1988

Leete E: The treatment of schizophrenia: a patient's perspective. Hosp Community Psychiatry 38:486–491, 1987

Individual Psychotherapy

Green H: I Never Promised You a Rose Garden. New York, Holt, Rinehart and Winston, 1964

Greenfeld D: The Psychotic Patient: Medication and Psychotherapy. New York, Free Press, 1985

Gunderson JG, Mosher LR (eds): Psychotherapy of Schizophrenia. New York, Jason Aronson, 1975

McGlashan TH: Intensive individual psychotherapy of schizophrenia: a review of techniques. Arch Gen Psychiatry 40:909–920, 1983

Family Involvement

Anderson CM, Hogarty GE, Reiss DJ: Family treatment of adult schizophrenic patients: a psycho-educational approach. Schizophr Bull 6:490–505, 1980

Falloon IRH, et al: Family Management of Schizophrenia: A Study of Clinical, Social, Family, and Economic Benefits. Baltimore, MD, Johns Hopkins University Press, 1985

Falloon IRH, Boyd JL, McGill CW: Family Care of Schizophrenia: A Problem-Solving Approach to the Treatment of Mental Illness. New York, Guilford, 1984

Group for the Advancement of Psychiatry: A Family Affair: Helping Families Cope With Mental Illness—A Guide for the Professions (GAP Rept No 119). New York, Brunner/Mazel, 1986

Hatfield AB: Families' Education in Mental Illness. Washington, DC, American Psychiatric Press, 1990

Johnson J: Hidden Victims. New York, Doubleday, 1988

Kanter J, Lamb HR, Loeper C: Expressed emotion in families: a critical review. Hosp Community Psychiatry 38:374–380, 1987

Lefley HP, Johnson DL (eds): Families as Allies in Treatment of the Mentally Ill: New Directions for Mental Health Professionals. Washington, DC, American Psychiatric Press, 1990

McGill CW, Lee E: Family psychoeducational intervention in the treatment of schizophrenia. Bull Menninger Clin 50:269–286, 1986

Seeman MV, Littman SK, Plummer E, et al: Living and Working With Schizophrenia. Toronto, University of Toronto Press, 1982

Terkelsen KG: Schizophrenia and the family, Part II: adverse effects of family therapy. Fam Process 22:191–200, 1983

Torrey EF: Surviving Schizophrenia: A Family Manual, Revised Edition. New York, Harper & Row, 1988

Walsh M: Schizophrenia: Straight Talk for Families and Friends. New York, William Morrow, 1986

Programs and Care Systems

Bachrach LL: Overview: model programs for chronic mental patients. Am J Psychiatry 137:1023–1031, 1980

Beard J, Propst R, Malamud T: The Fountain House model of psychiatric rehabilitation. Psychosocial Rehabilitation Journal 5:47–53, 1982

Shore MF, Gudeman JE (eds): Serving the Chronically Mentally Ill in an Urban Setting: The Massachusetts Mental Health Center Experience. New Directions for Mental Health Services No 39. San Francisco, CA, Jossey-Bass, 1988

Stein LI, Test MA: The Training in Community Living Model: A Decade of Experience. New Directions for Mental Health Services No 26. San Francisco, CA, Jossey-Bass, 1985

The Art of Medicating

Docherty JP, Fiester SJ: The therapeutic alliance and compliance with psychopharmacology, in Psychiatry Update: American Psychiatric Association Annual Review, Vol 4. Edited by Hales RE, Frances AJ. Washington, DC, American Psychiatric Press, 1985, pp 607–632

Marder SR, Swann E, Winslade WJ, et al: A study of medication refusal by involuntary psychiatric patients. Hosp Community Psychiatry 35:724–726, 1984

Van Putten T, Crumpton E, Yale C: Drug refusal in schizophrenia and the wish to be crazy. Arch Gen Psychiatry 33:1443–1446, 1976

Dual Diagnosis of Substance Abuse and Mental Illness

Drake RE, Osher FC, Wallach MA: Alcohol use and abuse in schizophrenia: a prospective community study. J Nerv Ment Dis 177:408–414, 1989

Lehman AF, Myers CP, Corty E: Assessment and classification of patients with psychiatric and substance abuse syndromes. Hosp Community Psychiatry 40:1019–1025, 1989

Lieberman JA, Bowers MB Jr: Substance abuse comorbidity in schizophrenia: editors' introduction. Schizophr Bull 16:29–30, 1990

Minkoff K: An integrated treatment model for dual diagnosis of psychosis and addiction. Hosp Community Psychiatry 40:1031–1036, 1989

Minkoff K, Drake RE (eds): Dual Diagnosis of Major Mental Illness and Substance Disorder. New Directions for Mental Health Services No 50. San Francisco, CA, Jossey-Bass, 1991

Osher FC, Kofoed LL: Treatment of patients with psychiatric and psychoactive substance abuse disorders. Hosp Community Psychiatry 40:1025–1030, 1989

Homeless Mentally Ill

Isaac RJ, Armat VC: Madness in the Streets: How Psychiatry and the Law Abandoned the Mentally Ill. New York, Free Press, 1990

Lamb HR (ed): The Homeless Mentally Ill: A Task Force Report of the American Psychiatric Association. Washington, DC, American Psychiatric Association, 1984

Lamb HR, Bachrach LL, Kass FI (eds): Treating the Homeless Mentally Ill: A Report of the Task Force on the Homeless Mentally Ill. Washington, DC, American Psychiatric Press, 1992

Talbott JA, Fine T: The homeless mentally ill, in The Homeless Mentally Ill. Chicago, IL, Mental Health Association of Chicago, 1986

GAP Committees and Membership

Committee on Adolescence

Warren J. Gadpaille, Denver, CO, *Chairperson*
Hector R. Bird, New York, NY
Ian A. Canino, New York, NY
Michael G. Kalogerakis, New York, NY
Paulina F. Kernberg, New York, NY
Clarice J. Kestenbaum, New York, NY
Richard C. Marohn, Chicago, IL
Silvio J. Onesti, Jr., Belmont, MA

Committee on Aging

Gene D. Cohen, Washington, DC, *Chairperson*
Karen Blank, West Hartford, CT
Eric D. Caine, Rochester, NY
Charles M. Gaitz, Houston, TX
Gary Gottlieb, Philadelphia, PA
Ira R. Katz, Philadelphia, PA
Andrew F. Leuchter, Los Angeles, CA
Gabe J. Maletta, Minneapolis, MN
Richard A. Margolin, Nashville, TN
Kenneth M. Sakauye, New Orleans, LA
Charles A. Shamoian, Larchmont, NY
F. Conyers Thompson, Jr., Atlanta, GA

Committee on Alcoholism and the Addictions

Joseph Westermeyer, Minneapolis, MN, *Chairperson*
Margaret H. Bean-Bayog, Lexington, MA
Susan J. Blumenthal, Washington, DC
Richard J. Frances, Newark, NJ
Marc Galanter, New York, NY
Earl A. Loomis, Jr., Augusta, GA

Sheldon I. Miller, Chicago, IL
Edgar P. Nace, Dallas, TX
Peter Steinglass, Washington, DC
John S. Tamerin, Greenwich, CT

Committee on Child Psychiatry

Peter E. Tanguay, Los Angeles, CA, *Chairperson*
James M. Bell, Canaan, NY
Mark Blotcky, Dallas, TX
Harlow Donald Dunton, New York, NY
Joseph Fischhoff, Detroit, MI
Joseph M. Green, Madison, WI
John F. McDermott, Jr., Honolulu, HI
David A. Mrazek, Denver, CO
Cynthia R. Pfeffer, White Plains, NY
John Schowalter, New Haven, CT
Theodore Shapiro, New York, NY
Leonore Terr, San Francisco, CA

Committee on College Students

Earle Silber, Chevy Chase, MD, *Chairperson*
Robert L. Arnstein, Hamden, CT
Varda Backus, La Jolla, CA
Harrison P. Eddy, New York, NY
Myron B. Liptzin, Chapel Hill, NC
Malkah Tolpin Notman, Brookline, MA
Gloria C. Onque, Pittsburgh, PA
Elizabeth Aub Reid, Cambridge, MA
Lorraine D. Siggins, New Haven, CT
Tom G. Stauffer, White Plains, NY

Committee on Cultural Psychiatry

Ezra Griffith, New Haven, CT, *Chairperson*
Edward Foulks, New Orleans, LA
Pedro Ruiz, Houston, TX
Ronald Wintrob, Providence, RI
Joe Yamamoto, Los Angeles, CA

Committee on the Family

Herta A. Guttman, Montreal, PQ, *Chairperson*

W. Robert Beavers, Dallas, TX
Ellen M. Berman, Merion, PA
Ira D. Glick, New York, NY
Frederick Gottlieb, Los Angeles, CA
Henry U. Grunebaum, Cambridge, MA
Judith Landau-Stanton, Rochester, NY
Ann L. Price, Avon, CT
Lyman C. Wynne, Rochester, NY

Committee on Government Policy

Roger Peele, Washington, DC, *Chairperson*
Thomas L. Clannon, San Francisco, CA
Naomi Heller, Washington, DC
John P. D. Shemo, Charlottesville, VA
William W. Van Stone, Washington, DC

Committee on Handicaps

William H. Sack, Portland, OR, *Chairperson*
Norman R. Bernstein, Cambridge, MA
Meyer S. Gunther, Wilmette, IL
Bryan King, Los Angeles, CA
Robert Nesheim, Duluth, MN
Betty J. Pfefferbaum, Norman, OK
William A. Sonis, Philadelphia, PA
Margaret L. Stuber, Los Angeles, CA
George Tarjan, Los Angeles, CA
Thomas G. Webster, Washington, DC
Henry H. Work, Bethesda, MD

Committee on Human Sexuality

Bertram H. Schaffner, New York, NY, *Chairperson*
Paul L. Adams, Galveston, TX
Debra Carter, Farmington, NM
Richard Friedman, New York, NY
Peggy Hanley-Hackenbruck, Portland, OR
Johanna A. Hoffman, Scottsdale, AZ
Joan A. Lang, Galveston, TX
Stuart E. Nichols, New York, NY
Harris B. Peck, New Rochelle, NY
Terry S. Stein, East Lansing, MI

Committee on International Relations

Vamik D. Volkan, Charlottesville, VA, *Chairperson*
Robert M. Dorn, El Macero, CA
John S. Kafka, Washington, DC
Otto F. Kernberg, White Plains, NY
Roy W. Menninger, Topeka, KS
Peter A. Olsson, Houston, TX
Rita R. Rogers, Palos Verdes Estates, CA
Stephen B. Shanfield, San Antonio, TX

Committee on Medical Education

Steven L. Dubovsky, Denver, CO, *Chairperson*
Leah Dickstein, Louisville, KY
Saul I. Harrison, Torrance, CA
David R. Hawkins, Chicago, IL
Jerry Kay, Dayton, OH
Harold I. Lief, Philadelphia, PA
Carol C. Nadelson, Boston, MA
Carolyn B. Robinowitz, Washington, DC
Stephen C. Scheiber, Deerfield, IL
Sidney L. Werkman, Washington, DC

Committee on Mental Health Services

W. Walter Menninger, Topeka, KS, *Chairperson*
Mary Jane England, Roseland, NJ
Robert O. Friedel, Richmond, VA
John M. Hamilton, Columbia, MD
Jose Maria Santiago, Tucson, AZ
Steven S. Sharfstein, Baltimore, MD
George F. Wilson, Somerville, NJ
Jack A. Wolford, Pittsburgh, PA

Committee on Planning and Communications

Robert W. Gibson, Towson, MD, *Chairperson*
Allan Beigel, Tucson, AZ
Doyle I. Carson, Dallas, TX
Paul J. Fink, Philadelphia, PA
Robert S. Garber, Longboat Key, FL
Richard K. Goodstein, Belle Mead, NJ
Harvey L. Ruben, New Haven, CT

Melvin Sabshin, Washington, DC
Michael R. Zales, Quechee, VT

Committee on Preventive Psychiatry

Naomi Rae-Grant, London, ON, *Chairperson*
Viola W. Bernard, New York, NY
Stephen Fleck, New Haven, CT
Brian J. McConville, Cincinnati, OH
David R. Offord, Hamilton, ON
Morton M. Silverman, Chicago, IL
Warren T. Vaughan, Jr., Portola Valley, CA
Ann Marie Wolf-Schatz, Conshohocken, PA

Committee on Psychiatry and the Community

H. Richard Lamb, Los Angeles, CA, *Chairperson*
Leona Bachrach, Gaithersburg, MD *(Consultant)*
Stephen Goldfinger, Boston, MA
David G. Greenfield, Guilford, CT
Kenneth Minkoff, Woburn, MA
John C. Nemiah, Hanover, NH
Becky Potter, Tucson, AZ
John J. Schwab, Louisville, KY
John A. Talbott, Baltimore, MD
Allan Tasman, Louisville, KY

Committee on Psychiatry and the Law

Joseph Satten, San Francisco, CA, *Chairperson*
J. Richard Ciccone, Rochester, NY
Carl P. Malmquist, Minneapolis, MN
Jeffrey Metzner, Denver, CO
Herbert C. Modlin, Topeka, KS
Jonas R. Rappeport, Baltimore, MD
Phillip J. Resnick, Cleveland, OH
Robert I. Simon, Bethesda, MD
William D. Weitzel, Lexington, KY

Committee on Psychiatry and Religion

Richard C. Lewis, New Haven, CT, *Chairperson*
Naleen N. Andrade, Honolulu, HI
Keith G. Meador, Nashville, TN

Abigail R. Ostow, Belmont, MA
Sally K. Severino, White Plains, NY
Clyde R. Snyder, Fayetteville, NC
Herzl Spiro, Milwaukee, WI
Edwin R. Wallace, IV, Augusta, GA

Committee on Psychiatry in Industry

David B. Robbins, Chappaqua, NY, *Chairperson*
Peter L. Brill, Radnor, PA
Barrie S. Greiff, Newton, MA
Duane Q. Hagen, St. Louis, MO
R. Edward Huffman, Asheville, NC
Robert Larsen, San Francisco, CA
David E. Morrison, Palatine, IL
Jay B. Rohrlich, New York, NY
Clarence J. Rowe, St. Paul, MN

Committee on Psychopathology

Robert A. Dorwart, Cambridge, MA, *Chairperson*
David A. Adler, Boston, MA
Jeffrey Berlant, Boise, ID
John P. Docherty, Nashua, NH
James M. Ellison, Watertown, MA
Howard H. Goldman, Potomac, MD
Kathleen A. Pajer, Pittsburgh, PA
Samuel G. Siris, Glen Oaks, NY

Committee on Public Education

Steven E. Katz, New York, NY, *Chairperson*
David Baron, Ambler, PA
Jack W. Bonner, III, Asheville, NC
Jeffrey L. Geller, Worcester, MA
Keith H. Johansen, Dallas, TX
Jeanne Leventhal, Hayward, CA
Elise K. Richman, Scarsdale, NY
Boris G. Rifkin, Branford, CT
Andrew E. Slaby, Summit, NJ
Robert A. Solow, Los Angeles, CA
Calvin R. Sumner, Buckhannon, WV

Committee on Research

Zebulon Taintor, New York, NY, *Chairperson*
Robert Cancro, New York, NY
John H. Greist, Madison, WI
Jerry M. Lewis, Dallas, TX
John G. Looney, Durham, NC
Sidney Malitz, New York, NY

Committee on Social Issues

Ian E. Alger, New York, NY, *Chairperson*
William R. Beardslee, Waban, MA
Roderic Gorney, Los Angeles, CA
Martha J. Kirkpatrick, Los Angeles, CA
Perry Ottenberg, Philadelphia, PA
Kendon W. Smith, Pearl River, NY

Committee on Therapeutic Care

William W. Richards, Anchorage, AK, *Chairperson*
Bernard Bandler, Cambridge, MA
Thomas E. Curtis, Chapel Hill, NC
Donald C. Fidler, Morgantown, WV
Donald W. Hammersley, Washington, DC
William B. Hunter, III, Albuquerque, NM
Roberto L. Jimenez, San Antonio, TX
Milton Kramer, Cincinnati, OH
John Lipkin, Perry Point, MA
Theodore Nadelson, Jamaica Plain, MA

Committee on Therapy

Jules R. Bemporad, White Plains, NY, *Chairperson*
Gerald Adler, Boston, MA
Eugene B. Feigelson, Brooklyn, NY
Robert Michels, New York, NY
Andrew P. Morrison, Cambridge, MA
William C. Offenkrantz, Scottsdale, AZ
Allan D. Rosenblatt, La Jolla, CA

GINSBURG FELLOWS

Michael R. Arambula, Chicago, IL *(Committee on Government Policy)*
B. James Bennett, Dallas, TX *(Committee on Adolescence)*
Deborah L. Cabaniss, New York, NY *(Committee on Medical Education)*
Laura J. Dalheim, Barrington, RI *(Committee on Therapeutic Care)*
Alex R. Demac, New Haven, CT *(Committee on Public Education)*
Hinda F. Dubin, Baltimore, MD *(Committee on Psychiatry and Religion)*
James R. Dumerauf, Waukesha, WI *(Committee on Handicaps)*
Denise M. Heebink, New York, NY *(Committee on International Relations)*
Patricia L. Hough, Augusta, GA *(Committee on Social Issues)*
Jonathan House, New York, NY *(Committee on Therapy)*
David J. Kapley, Chapel Hill, NC *(Committee on Psychiatry and the Law)*
Shitij Kapur, Pittsburgh, PA *(Committee on Psychopathology)*
Debra F. Kirsch, Houston, TX *(Committee on Alcoholism and the Addictions)*
Laura W. Lane, Albuquerque, NM *(Committee on Preventive Psychiatry)*
Constantine G. Lyketsos, Baltimore, MD *(Committee on Research)*
Elizabeth A. Murphy, Boston, MA *(Committee on Cultural Psychiatry)*
Michel Paradis, Montreal, PQ *(Committee on Psychiatry in Industry)*
Linda M. Peterson, Owings Mills, MD *(Committee on Psychiatry and the Community)*
Anthony Poehailos, Charlottesville, VA *(Committee on Child Psychiatry)*
Rachel G. Seidel, Belmont, MA *(Committee on Planning and Communications)*
Rita A. Shaughnessy, Oak Park, IL *(Committee on Mental Health Services)*
Joseph A. Shrand, West Simsbury, CT *(Committee on the Family)*
Grace C. Vigilante, New Orleans, LA *(Committee on College Students)*
Susan L. Warren, Somerville, MA *(Committee on Aging)*
Gwen L. Zornberg, Belmont, MA *(Committee on Human Sexuality)*

Contributing Members

Gene Abroms, Ardmore, PA
Carlos C. Alden, Jr., Buffalo, NY
Kenneth Z. Altshuler, Dallas, TX
Francis F. Barnes, Washington, DC
Spencer Bayles, Houston, TX
C. Christian Beels, New York, NY
Elissa P. Benedek, Ann Arbor, MI
Sidney Berman, Washington, DC
Renee L. Binder, San Francisco, CA
H. Keith H. Brodie, Durham, NC
Charles M. Bryant, San Francisco, CA
Ewald W. Busse, Durham, NC
Robert N. Butler, New York, NY
Eugene M. Caffey, Jr., Bowie, MD
Robert J. Campbell, New York, NY
James P. Cattell, San Diego, CA
Ian L.W. Clancey, Maitland, ON
Sanford I. Cohen, Coral Gables, FL
Lee Combrinck-Graham, Evanston, IL
Charles M. Culver, Hanover, NH
Robert E. Drake, Hanover, NH
James S. Eaton, Jr., Washington, DC
Lloyd C. Elam, Nashville, TN
Joseph T. English, New York, NY
Sherman C. Feinstein, Highland Park, IL
Archie R. Foley, New York, NY
Sidney Furst, Bronx, NY
Henry J. Gault, Highland Park, IL
Judith H. Gold, Halifax, NS
Alexander Gralnick, Port Chester, NY
Milton Greenblatt, Sylmar, CA
Lawrence F. Greenleigh, Los Angeles, CA
Stanley I. Greenspan, Bethesda, MD
Jon E. Gudeman, Milwaukee, WI
Stanley Hammons, Lexington, KY
William Hetznecker, Merion Station, PA
J. Cotter Hirschberg, Topeka, KS
Johanna A. Hoffman, Scottsdale, AZ
Jay Katz, New Haven, CT
Edward J. Khantzian, Haverhill, MA
James A. Knight, New Orleans, LA

Othilda M. Krug, Cincinnati, OH
Anthony F. Lehman, Baltimore, MD
Alan I. Levenson, Tucson, AZ
Ruth W. Lidz, Woodbridge, CT
Orlando B. Lightfoot, Boston, MA
Norman L. Loux, Sellersville, PA
Albert J. Lubin, Woodside, CA
John Mack, Chestnut Hill, MA
John A. MacLeod, Cincinnati, OH
Charles A. Malone, Barrington, RI
Peter A. Martin, Lake Orion, MI
Ake Mattsson, Greenville, NC
Alan A. McLean, Gig Harbor, WA
David Mendell, Houston, TX
Mary E. Mercer, Nyack, NY
Derek Miller, Chicago, IL
Steven M. Mirin, Belmont, MA
Richard D. Morrill, Boston, MA
Robert J. Nathan, Philadelphia, PA
Joseph D. Noshpitz, Washington, DC
Mortimer Ostow, Bronx, NY
Bernard L. Pacella, New York, NY
Herbert Pardes, New York, NY
Norman L. Paul, Lexington, MA
Marvin E. Perkins, Salem, VA
George H. Pollock, Chicago, IL
Becky Potter, Tucson, AZ
David N. Ratnavale, Bethesda, MD
Richard E. Renneker, Pacific Palisades, CA
W. Donald Ross, Cincinnati, OH
Loren Roth, Pittsburgh, PA
Donald J. Scherl, Brooklyn, NY
Charles Shagass, Philadelphia, PA
Miles F. Shore, Boston, MA
Albert J. Silverman, Ann Arbor, MI
Benson R. Snyder, Cambridge, MA
David A. Soskis, Bala Cynwyd, PA
Jeffrey L. Speller, Cambridge, MA
Jeanne Spurlock, Washington, DC
Brandt F. Steele, Denver, CO
Alan A. Stone, Cambridge, MA
Perry C. Talkington, Dallas, TX
John Talbott, Baltimore, MD

Bryce Templeton, Philadelphia, PA
Prescott W. Thompson, Portland, OR
John A. Turner, San Francisco, CA
Gene L. Usdin, New Orleans, LA
Kenneth N. Vogtsberger, San Antonio, TX
Andrew S. Watson, Ann Arbor, MI
Joseph B. Wheelwright, Kentfield, CA
Robert L. Williams, Houston, TX
Paul Tyler Wilson, Bethesda, MD
Sherwyn M. Woods, Los Angeles, CA
Kent A. Zimmerman, Menlo Park, CA
Howard Zonana, New Haven, CT

Life Members

C. Knight Aldrich, Charlottesville, VA
Robert L. Arnstein, Hamden, CT
Bernard Bandler, Cambridge, MA
Walter E. Barton, Hartland, VT
Viola W. Bernard, New York, NY
Henry W. Brosin, Tucson, AZ
John Donnelly, Hartford, CT
Merrill T. Eaton, Omaha, NE
O. Spurgeon English, Narberth, PA
Stephen Fleck, New Haven, CT
Jerome Frank, Baltimore, MD
Robert S. Garber, Longboat Key, FL
Robert I. Gibson, Towson, MD
Margaret M. Lawrence, Pomona, NY
Jerry M. Lewis, Dallas, TX
Harold I. Lief, Philadelphia, PA
Judd Marmor, Los Angeles, CA
Herbert C. Modlin, Topeka, KS
John C. Nemiah, Hanover, NH
William C. Offenkrantz, Scottsdale, AZ
Mabel Ross, Sun City, AZ
Julius Schreiber, Washington, DC
Robert E. Switzer, Dunn Loring, VA
Jack A. Wolford, Pittsburgh, PA
Henry H. Work, Bethesda, MD

*Leo H. Bartemeier 1963–65
Robert S. Garber 1965–67
Herbert C. Modlin 1967–69
John Donnelly 1969–71
George Tarjan 1971–73
Judd Marmor 1973–75
John C. Nemiah 1975–77
Jack A. Wolford 1977–79
Robert W. Gibson 1979–81
*Jack Weinberg 1981–82
Henry H. Work 1982–85
Michael R. Zales 1985–87
Jerry M. Lewis 1987–89
Carolyn B. Robinowitz 1989–91

PUBLICATIONS BOARD

Chairperson
C. Knight Aldrich
905 Cottage Lane
Charlottesville, VA 22903

Robert L. Arnstein
Mark Blotcky
Ezra Griffith
Steve Katz
W. Walter Menninger

Consultants
John C. Nemiah
Henry H. Work

Ex-Officio
Allan Beigel
Carolyn B. Robinowitz

CONTRIBUTORS

Abbott Laboratories
American Charitable Fund
Dr. and Mrs. Richard Aron

---

*Deceased.

Mr. Robert C. Baker
Bristol-Myers Squibb Co.
Maurice Falk Medical Fund
Mrs. Carol Gold
Edith F. Goldensohn
Grove Foundation, Inc.
Miss Gayle Groves
Ittleson Foundation, Inc.
Mr. Barry Jacobson
Mrs. Allan H. Kalmus
Marion E. Kenworthy–Sarah H. Swift Foundation, Inc.
Mr. Larry Korman
McNeil Pharmaceutical
Murel Foundation
Phillips Foundation
Sandoz Corporation
Smith Kline Beckman Corporation
Tappanz Foundation, Inc.
The Upjohn Company
van Ameringen Foundation, Inc.
Wyeth-Ayerst Laboratories
Mr. and Mrs. William A. Zales

Index of Continuing Case Examples

Index

Note: Page numbers in **boldface** type refer to tables.